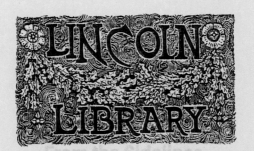
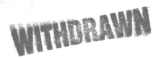

"This is the story of a woman with a bad heart who was able to overcome all challenges with tenacity and a good heart. Emily Falcon is a gifted storyteller. The story is packed with action. It is a reminder to value every single day, hour, minute."
—Dr. Marius Stan, scientist, author, and actor (*Breaking Bad*)

"Perseverance, determination, and a positive attitude toward oneself and the ability to seize opportunity are just a few takeaways from Emily's personal and heartwarming story."
—Jack Fleming, President and CEO, Boston Athletic Association

"Emily takes the reader into her tumultuous health journey, which placed her on the sidelines. It culminates in her ability to move from the sidelines into the path of active participation. I shed tears when she described her many experiences with failed cardioversions and ablations and could not begin to imagine the anxiety and frustration that she endured. I rejoice with her now that she can move from the sidelines to the finish line of almost everything."
—Daphne Davis-Patrick, DNP, Author, Educator, Inspirational Speaker

"A powerful, personal story of a woman fighting for independence and happiness. It's difficult to talk openly about one's fears and self-conscious feelings. Emily lets us know exactly what she was feeling. She lets us inside the experience of living with chronic illness."
—Frank Jaworski, CRNA, father to an adult born with congenital heart disease (CHD)

"I love the uplifting message of this book. It's so good to have this out there for people who feel their problems are just too much to overcome. Emily is very relatable to anyone who's struggled with long-term health issues."
—Hope Angelina, author, *The Story of Hope: A Mother and Transdaughter's Odyssey of Rediscovery,* to be published in 2024; adult with CHD

"As a heart patient myself, I felt like I was gaining a friend while reading Emily's book. She described the life and emotions of a heart warrior so well! I was very touched by Emily's story."
—Lauren Elizabeth, author, *Lessons from a Broken Heart,* to be published in 2024; graphic designer; adult with CHD

"This is a story of a woman and her team of caregivers' amazing journey of multiple medical challenges and her successes over them. Emily is a role model for all who face and overcome challenges. Having cared for hundreds of adults with CHD I still found the final race description to be very impactful and I will admit it brought me to tears."
—Disty Pearson, PA-C

From the Sidelines to the Finish Line

A Chronic Illness Survivor's Challenges and Everyday Triumphs

Emily Falcon

Baby Hearts Press
Temple, Texas

The names of some people in the book have been changed but not places. The author has tried to recreate events, locales, and conversations from her memories of them.

This book is not intended or implied to be a substitute for professional medical advice, diagnosis, or treatment. Consequently, this book should not be used to define medical treatment for any child or adult. Please consult your doctor for treatment of your particular condition. The purpose of this book is to inspire others. The author and Don't Waste A Second Press/Baby Hearts Press shall have neither liability nor responsibility to any person or entity with respect to any loss or damage caused, or alleged to be caused, directly or indirectly, by the information contained in this book.

Publisher's Cataloging-in-Publication Data

Names: Falcon, Emily, author.

Title: From the sidelines to the finish line : a chronic illness survivor's challenges and everyday triumphs / Emily Falcon

Description: Temple, TX : Baby Hearts Press, 2023

Summary: A memoir about chronic illnesses including a congenital cardiac condition and glaucoma, a story of survival.

Identifiers:
LCCN 2023911834 I ISBN 9780965250887 (pbk.) I ISBN 9780965250894 (ebook)

Subjects:
LCSH: 1. Falcon, Emily. 2. Chronic diseases—Patients—United States—Biography. 3. Heart—Surgery—Patients—United States—Biography

LCGFT: Autobiographies

BISAC: BIOGRAPHY & AUTOBIOGRAPHY / Medical. HEALTH & FITNESS / Physical Impairments. I SELF-HELP / Motivational & Inspirational.

Classification: LCC: PS3606.A42298 F76 2023 I DDC 811.6--dc22

Library of Congress Cataloging in Publication information is on file.

First printing 2023 in United States

Publisher: Don't Waste A Second Press

Publishing imprint:
Baby Hearts Press, LLC
3910 Sierra Blanca Blvd., Temple, TX 76502-1662 U.S.A.
babyheartspress@gmail.com
babyheartspress.com/emily-falcon

Contents

Foreword

My brother Rick had cerebral palsy and was a nonspeaking quadriplegic. To communicate he had to type his messages out one letter at a time. One day he asked our father, "Can I run in a race?" and Dad said, "Yes you can!" When they got home from the race Rick wrote on his computer, "Dad, when I am running it feels like my disability disappears." Dad was hooked, and he had a custom racing chair built in order for them to participate in races. My father, Dick Hoyt, and my brother, Rick, ran the Boston Marathon together thirty-two times. They were known as Team Hoyt, a father-son duo who advocated for people living with disabilities.

The Hoyt Foundation was formed in 1989 and aspires to build the individual character, self-confidence, and self-esteem of America's disabled young people through inclusion in all facets of daily life. We educate the public about disability awareness and promote the Team Hoyt motto, "Yes You Can."

Emily Falcon makes our mission a reality. One of her mottoes is, "Just Try," and ours, "Yes You Can," shine throughout this book. Falcon tells a stranger, "If I can do it, you can too!" She participates in challenges even when the task might seem insurmountable. Her story enables readers to realize their own potential. Whether it's going on a walk or running in a race, Falcon demonstrates believing in yourself and never giving up.

Her resilience and determination have allowed her to become a strong athlete, something no one thought was possible. Her obstacles and triumphs are relatable to anyone who has faced and wants to overcome hardships. The advice she gives will make you want to get out there and participate!

Team Hoyt completed more than 1,100 races together. Falcon's race total might someday match my father's and brother's with her strong determination. She will motivate you to achieve your dreams and make the impossible possible because, yes, you can!

Russ Hoyt
President & CEO
The Hoyt Foundation
teamhoyt.com

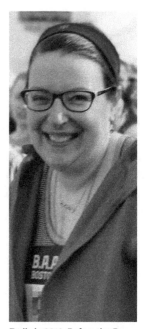

Emily in 2018, Before the Race

Prologue

In April 2018, I blended into a crowd of 10,000 athletes eager to hear the starting gun for the 5K race to begin. Smoothing out my running leggings and tank top, and glancing down at my runner's bib with my number, I glimpsed my pink and purple chest scar shining brightly. The scar came from my open-heart surgery eight months prior. None of the other participants knew that I had a heart condition or that I had overcome thirty-five years of obstacles to take part in this race. Like everyone else, I was anxious and ready to start running, hoping to do my best.

I had never participated in gym class or sports because of my heart condition, so this was a first for me. In the past, even a set of stairs or an incline could leave me breathless on some days. In the previous few decades of my life, I could never even have contemplated joining an athletic event because I wasn't physically ready to meet the challenge, but I was now attempting it. Trying not to become overwhelmed thinking about what I hoped to accomplish with my newly changed body, I heard the starting gun, and the race commenced.

The elite runners took off. Eventually it was my turn to advance to the starting line, away from my family. As I walked ahead, I took in my surroundings, hearing the cheers of the crowd and seeing the tall Boston skyscrapers shining radiantly against the sunny blue sky. Everything was full of promise. The buildings reflected the green grass of Boston Common and the blur of athletes and spectators. I began to feel more excited than anxious. As I went around the last corner on Beacon Street before the starting line, I saw my family in the crowd. We waved goodbye. Turning on my music playlist, I ran over the starting line and began ...

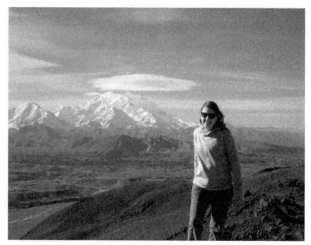

Emily and Mt. Denali (September 13, 2018)

Introduction

What is it like to experience the strength and vitality of youth for the first time at age thirty-five? This is a story of my personal "Benjamin Button" journey. In F. Scott Fitzgerald's short story "The Curious Case of Benjamin Button," Benjamin is born an old man and experiences life in reverse, taking on new abilities as he becomes younger. In my case, as a result of a life-altering surgery, my abilities continue to develop, and I feel younger and more fit every day.

I went from being unable to run more than a few yards to developing as an athlete who participated in my first athletic event, a 5K race, just eight months after open-heart surgery. I chose to move away from the comfort of my medical team and family in Boston to Alaska, where physical challenges were part of everyday life. Whether hiking in Denali National Park, getting lost in the woods, or whitewater rafting in freezing rapids, I found my endurance tested in ways it had never been previously.

I have never had a normal life. At seven weeks old, in 1982, I had a heart attack that destroyed forty percent of the left side of my heart. My heart condition forever altered the course of my life and led to two open-heart surgeries, one at age six and another at age thirty-five.

A little over a year after my second surgery, my cardiac surgeon gave a presentation that featured my medical journey. After the talk, many audience members came up to me and told me they were inspired by my story. I didn't understand why, or why they called me a hero. I felt like all I had done was go on living and trying, which I did not feel made me stand out. One audience member shared her fears and hesitation about trying to go on a hike. I responded, "If I can do it, you can too!" Taken aback for a moment, she then agreed to give hiking a try. For the first time, I realized how my story could inspire others.

This book is about my experiences and how I have felt leading a life with complex, chronic medical issues. Unlike many survivors who have experienced sudden traumatic illness or accidents that forced them to live with newly acquired limitations, I have an uncommon perspective, from both a child's and an adult's viewpoint, because I have experienced a rare and chronic illness from birth.

At times, it might seem discouraging to read about everything I went through, and it might seem as if life will never improve, but it does. The skills and knowledge of my medical team, endless support from my family, and my own dogged perseverance enabled me to live a life no one ever dreamed was possible. No one and nothing, least of all my body, is holding me back anymore. I want to fully explore my abilities after a lifetime of restrictions and live my motto to the fullest: "Don't waste a second." By sharing aspects of my journey, I hope my insights can encourage people who doubt their own resilience.

Today, I live in a different world, one that is full of potential. My wish is to show people who hold back from experiences that maybe they can make a different choice. People with chronic illness can be inspired and learn to advocate for themselves. They can appreciate their level of health and not take it for granted. All opportunities, both big and small, should be embraced. Never waste a moment and don't let life pass you by!

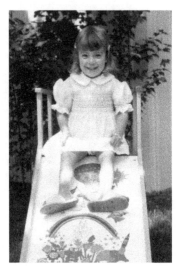

Emily, Third Birthday (July 1985)

The History of Emily

"She's here!" Dad exuberantly told his parents-in-law over the phone in late July 1982.* "She's five pounds, seven ounces, and everything's perfect."

"You're joking, that can't be. The baby's not due for thirty more days."

"It's true. Now you'll have to come to Boston to meet her."

After a few days in the hospital, when Mom had recuperated from her cesarean section, we were ready to go home.

"What will she wear to go home?" Dad asked Mom as he unpacked a small suitcase with some onesies.

"We only have a few choices since Emily's small and we haven't gone shopping yet. What about this white onesie?" On it, blue and yellow turtles with racer helmets were speeding along on fast wheels, and orange bears with yellow headphones listened to music.

"That looks good and we have to get some supplies," Dad replied.

Soon my parents adjusted to our new lives together. Mom worked as a copywriter and had her baby shower at her office the week prior to my arrival. Dad was an electrical engineer and is from the Midwest, which you wouldn't notice until he says things like "Q-pon" instead of "coupon."

---

*My dad kept a detailed diary that cataloged important events and milestones in my life. His account and recollections are used here to help tell my story, interspersed with my memories and my mom's.

On a sunny September day, when I was seven and half weeks old, my parents took me to the beach to hear ocean waves for the first time and to see the sandy shores of Nantasket Beach. I was unable to enjoy the seagulls and warm weather.

"Why won't she stop crying?" Mom asked, exasperated. "I've tried feeding her, and she won't drink."

Dad stared at me in confusion. "Maybe she has a cold?"

My parents called my pediatrician, who said calmly, "Don't worry. Babies often cry. No need to come in for an exam."

The next day, Mom called the pediatrician again. "She's still not drinking and now she's vomited."

"Okay, bring her in to see me." When we got there, he listened to my heart and said to Mom, "Go to Massachusetts General Hospital *immediately*!"

Mom quickly drove into Boston and parked in front of the hospital, MGH, in the ambulance bay and rushed me inside. I was admitted to the Pediatric Intensive Care Unit (PICU), since the doctors knew something was wrong with my heart. On about the fourth day they confirmed that I'd had a heart attack.

The doctors diagnosed me with anomalous origin of the left coronary artery from the pulmonary artery (ALCAPA), after a period of testing in the PICU. This means my left coronary artery*, which carries blood to the heart muscle, arose from the pulmonary artery instead of the aorta. This prevented my heart's blood supply from having sufficient oxygen and blood pressure, resulting in my heart attack. My condition is not inherited; rather it occurs during fetal development. I also had mitral valve regurgitation, meaning my valve leaked and blood went in the wrong direction. The valve had been fine before the heart attack, when it was damaged. I survived my heart attack because of the good care I received in the hospital and because my body created extra pathways, also known

---

*See the Medical Glossary at the end of the book for definitions.

as collateral arteries, to feed blood to the weaker side. Without those things, I never would have survived.

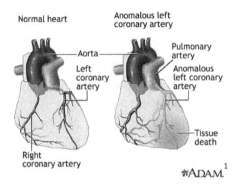

If I had been born even thirty years earlier, I would have had scarce options, but by the 1980s, although there was little compared to what there is today, technology had advanced enough to offer treatment options for children.

After my heart attack and initial diagnosis, I remained in the hospital, as I was too ill to return home. Mom stopped breastfeeding me soon after I was admitted, because it was too hard.

"Not many children survive this cardiac condition into adulthood," my doctor gently told my parents. Questioning my future and hoping for the best, everyone silently looked at me in the crib, intubated on a respirator to help me breathe, fed through an IV (intravenous transmission of medication or food), listening to the machines beeping and keeping me alive. The internet did not exist yet, and my parents had no family medical history that gave them prior knowledge about cardiac care or how to navigate life with a child in the hospital.

In the 1980s, it was rare to diagnose my condition and to find hospitals or cardiologists with experience treating it. Congenital heart defects are the most common type of birth defect in the United States, affecting about one in 100 babies,[2] and ALCAPA occurs

0.25–0.5 percent[3] of the time, with an overall prevalence rate of one out of every 300,000 births.

My doctors figured things out as they went along with no clear guidelines or treatment manual, using the knowledge they had at the time and consulting with other physicians. The doctors considered transferring me to Boston Children's Hospital, where the cardiologists consulted wanted to perform my corrective surgery right away. My cardiologist at MGH advocated waiting until my heart grew larger and stronger. My parents agreed this was the best option, so I stayed a patient of MGH, where they provided medications, testing, and monitoring. Some days my health was precarious. Mom said, "During the months at MGH we were told that each hour that you lived was a good hour."

Currently, there are clearer treatment plans and prognoses for people with ALCAPA, with basic information readily available. Data now suggests that when ALCAPA is untreated, approximately ninety percent of babies die within the first year of life.[4] Children who are diagnosed and treated now, with more experienced doctors and clinics in the United States, mostly grow up to live a normal life.[5]

Autumn 1982

Little milestones during this trying time were a huge victory. Almost a month after admission, my doctors took me off the respirator and Dad wrote in his diary, "Emily gets her IVs out and starts to eat milk, then powdered bananas, then peaches!" A few days later, "Emily can be carried for a walk down the hall!" Since I almost died, every little new thing I did became a big deal. The doctors asked Mom to participate in some experiments to learn more about infant cardiac patients. Each time she left the room, my heart rate rose, and it lowered upon her return.

A month later, the doctors moved me out of the PICU to the Intermediate Care Unit (IMCU), which meant my health was improving. When I was taken out of my room for tests, I enjoyed a painting on the ceiling in the hallway of the dwarfs from *Snow White and the Seven Dwarfs*. Dad pointed at all the dwarfs and I laughed, looking at Dopey in his long, olive green dress and cone-shaped blue hat.

During a brisk autumn week, almost two months after the warm beach weekend and my hospital admission, my parents brought me home. They gave me numerous medications and we had regular trips to doctors and occasional Emergency Room (ER) visits. Mom took care of me, not returning to work after I was diagnosed, realizing that I needed her care full-time. I lived in congestive heart failure. This meant that my heart couldn't pump blood efficiently to get rid of fluid, so I couldn't add more liquid to my diet. I quickly commenced eating solid food that Mom made from scratch, much earlier than other infants. My fluid intake was limited to four ounces a day and after some improvement went up to six ounces per day, while an average baby might drink that amount at each feeding.

Spring and Summer 1983

For the first time, in early March, the electrocardiogram (EKG) showed a dramatic improvement in the electrical activity in my heart. My parents celebrated my first birthday in July, and Dad wrote in his journal, "She made it!" The doctor's care plan was working.

Three months later, the doctor performed an echocardiogram ("echo") to view the inside structures and blood flow of my heart via ultrasound. After the test, my pediatric cardiologist, Dr. Gold, called my parents with the results. "The infarct, or dead tissue resulting from Emily's heart attack, is starting to gradually become a smaller part of the heart as the healthy parts of the heart continue to grow ... but, her other problem, the mitral valve regurgitation, is not improving and continues to leak. We'll continue to monitor it."

July 1984

From the time I was a baby, my parents supervised my activity. They were happy I could play quietly with my stuffed animals.

"There she goes with Teddy," Dad smiled. "You might have to wash him soon so we can tell he's a polar bear again!"

Mom asked me, "Why aren't you eating, Emily?"

"Teddy's hungry," I said, feeding him some food before eating myself.

Teddy helped me celebrate my second birthday. I blew out the candles and shared some cake with him.

A few days later, Mom asked Dad, "Your boss gave you the day off for Emily's doctor's appointment, right?"

"Yes, of course. If she might have to have the surgery soon, I can't miss that."

When I got home from Dr. Gold's, I was playing on the floor with my dolls and Dad knelt down beside me with batteries to put into my broken toy.

"Emily, your toy's broken. Who can fix this?"

"Dr. Gold!" I announced. Even at a very young age, I believed my cardiologist could make everything better.

A few weeks later, Mom spoke to Dr. Gold on the phone while I played on the floor in the kitchen.

"I have good news!" he said. "The consensus amongst my colleagues and me is to adjust Emily's medications. Let's let her grow bigger before we operate on her heart. She's doing well and I'd love to wait as long as we can. That will reduce the likelihood of us needing to perform a second surgery later to accommodate her growing heart."

August 1987

I had a live-in babysitter, Marty, over the summer. She was there to care for me and help out around the house, since Mom was expecting a baby. At the end of August, Marty and I were eating lunch in the living room when the phone rang. Excitedly, I rushed toward the kitchen.

"You're a big sister now!" Dad said.

Twirling the phone cord around my finger, I pressed the phone closer to my ear.

"Mom's fine. I'll be home tonight. You can meet your baby sister, Sam, soon."

I squealed and jumped up and down with excitement.

Summer 1988

I got off the bus on my last day of kindergarten to find Sam and Mom were waiting for me.

"Happy last day of school!" Mom said.

We walked across the street to the car.

"We can go out to Friendly's to celebrate. Sam will get to try her first ice cream now that she's almost one."

"I can't wait!" I squeezed Sam's hand. "You can have some of my bubblegum ice cream!"

When we got home from Friendly's, Dad had already come home and changed out of his work clothes.

"Dr. Gold called," Mom told him. "They want Emily to have a cardiac catheterization so the doctors can determine if it's time for her open-heart surgery."

"I hope this time the dye will show something good … It's going to be okay," Dad reassured her.

On the day of the test, I sat on the floor of Sam's room brushing her curly hair. "I'm going to the hospital," I told her while selecting a blue barrette and snapping it in place.

Sam smiled at me and grabbed a green barrette and put it in her mouth.

"I'm going for a 'poke, poke' but I'll be asleep." I took the barrette out of Sam's mouth.

Grandma came into the room and took Sam into her arms and waved goodbye as we left for the hospital.

My roommate in the hospital was a baby less than a year old who slept in a silver steel crib in one corner of our room. During my recovery, I sat with him when he cried and held his hand. "Don't worry, you'll get better and go home. It won't hurt much longer."

A few days later when it was time for me to return home, the baby's mother patted my shoulder and said, "Thank you so much for helping my son. Here's a gift for you." She handed me a *Sesame Street*–themed activity book. On the ride home I happily flipped through the pages.

Fall 1988

Two months after my hospital stay my aunt came from California to visit the family.

"We'll be home soon," Mom told Auntie. "Echoes only take about an hour and with the drive we'll be home by dinner time."

"Let's go, Emily," Dad said as he handed Sam to Auntie. "We're going to the hospital again."

"Bye-bye, Sam!" I said after pulling her curl straight and letting it bounce back into place to make her laugh.

"Do you think we'll see Nurse Robin again?" I asked Mom in the car.

"No, she works on the kids' floor where you had your poke, poke. We're just going in for a test this time."

At the hospital, Nurse Robin surprised us as we signed into the echo lab.

"I have a present for you!" she said, handing me a wrapped rectangular box.

Underneath the wrapping paper was a Barbie doll. She had blonde hair, a sky-blue spaghetti-strap tank top, and a long white-and-blue skirt.

I squealed in delight, "I don't have any Barbies at home."

I named my favorite doll Robin (not a Barbie) after my favorite nurse. From then on whenever I had a test at the hospital, I often brought my treasured confidante along. At one chest X-ray, I carried Robin with me. The technician took an X-ray of Robin, which showed her empty inside. I brought it in to show and tell at school.

A few weeks after the X-ray Sam and I both contracted a virus. She got better in a few days, but I was still sick.

Mom called the nurse to ask how to help me.

The nurse replied, "It's cold-and-flu season now that it's the middle of October, so it's not surprising both Sam and Emily would be sick. Since Emily's still sick, while Sam has already recovered, you'd better bring her in."

Mom hung up the phone and checked in on Sam and me in the living room. I was curled up on the couch watching *DuckTales,* enjoying the time away from school. Sam was in her playpen, playing with her toys.

Mom returned to the kitchen and dialed Dad's work number. "The nurse said I need to bring Emily to the hospital."

"Aren't there any medications we can give her?"

"No, they're afraid of how they will affect her heart. ... Okay, see you there." She hung up.

"Emily, we need to go to the hospital," Mom said as she put Sam's diaper bag by the front door. She turned off the television. "Time to get you dressed."

"Okay," I said, and got up to do what she asked.

At the hospital, Mom completed check-in paperwork while balancing Sam on her hip.

The nurse guided us to a gurney in the hallway, saying, "Let's keep Emily away from the sicker patients."

"Up you go!" said a man in scrubs as he lifted me onto the gurney.

Mom gave me some M&M's while we were alone waiting. Tearing open the brown bag, I decided the green ones were my favorite. With green-coated fingers, I slowly ate one M&M after another while waiting for tests. Later that day, I settled into my room. Tired from all the tests and feeling poorly, I lay down.

Peeking her head into my room a nurse said, "Visiting hours are over."

"We'll be back tomorrow," Mom said as she turned to leave.

I slept like a log. My parents came to visit me the next day. "The doctor thinks you can go home tomorrow," Dad said.

"Yay," I said.

I dozed off on the ride home. In the afternoon, I overheard Mom talking to my teacher on the phone. "She can only come back to school part time for three weeks."

Two weeks later, on Halloween night, I wore a white scarf draped in my hair with gold sequins shaped like leaves dangling across my forehead, a pink tunic, large silver hoop clip-on earrings, and multicolored plastic bracelets. I got into my father's silver Honda Accord and we drove the short distance from house to house to trick or treat.

Striding up the walkways of the neighbor's homes in the crisp fall air to ring the doorbells and eagerly anticipate my treats was taxing, and I didn't make it to many houses.

"Next fall you'll get your flu shot earlier and maybe you won't get as many viruses," Dad said. "Hopefully you can go trick-or-treating at more houses next year."

When we got home, Mom got me ready for bed.

"I don't want a flu shot. I hate needles," I told Mom.

"I know, Emily, but would you rather have one shot, or spend three weeks in the hospital with an IV suffering from the flu?" my mother asked.

As Thanksgiving drew nearer, I realized one of my teeth was loose and was ready to fall out. When I pushed at it with my tongue it started to bleed. Standing next to Mom who was seated on the couch at about the same height as me, I stamped my feet. "No, don't make me do it," I sobbed. "I can't take it out!" My tears flowed freely as I tasted the bitter warm blood in my mouth.

Mom sternly responded, "You have to do it. I can't do it for you. I know you're not used to normal scrapes and bruises because you don't go outside to play, but this is a normal part of being a kid."

I'll have to go to the hospital because I'm bleeding. I'm keeping this tooth in as long as I can. I rocked the tooth that was hanging on by a thread, back and forth, for as long as I could, stubbornly dragging out the process. It finally detached without any pain, and the light bleeding stopped. The entire removal took from afternoon until sundown.

When Dad came home from work, I proudly showed him the tooth with a massive smile on my face. *I didn't even have to go to the hospital.* "The tooth fairy's coming tonight!"

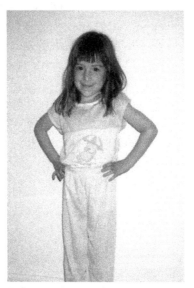

Emily, Age 5 (May 1988)

The First Surgery

As I was sitting in the living room playing with my dolls, home from school for a snow day, I asked Mom, "Why can't the doctors fix what's wrong with my heart?"

Surprised, Mom looked up from the book she was reading. "The doctors plan to repair your heart soon," she said.

Picking up Robin, I walked to my bedroom and looked at the American Heart Association poster on my wall. It had a cartoon boy and his circulatory system. I wanted to understand how my heart worked. Nobody ever talked to me about my body or my heart condition. I stared at the poster and I wished I could understand what made my heart different and how it could be fixed.

March 26, 1989
On the Sunday before my surgery, Grandma drove up from Connecticut.

"Sam needs her lunch at 12," Mom said to Grandma. "Emily has to go in for two days of presurgery testing. We'll be home tonight. Dr. Gold's meeting us, so we have to go now."

Dad said, "Emily, let me help you put on your jacket." My parents live in a suburb of Boston, about a thirty-minute drive away from the hospital. Walking toward the car, I was excited by the attention my parents gave me. I reached for the handle of the door to the back seat as I normally would, but my parents stopped me. "Sit in the front seat between us."

Something special's happening if I get to sit here! As we drove past our white house and the budding trees in the yard, I didn't realize it at the time, but that could have been our last car ride together.

The next two days were a blur of blood tests, EKGs, and other tests. Nurses bustled in and out of my room and my parents stayed with me during the day.

On Tuesday morning, the anesthesiologist walked into my room. "I'm going to give you some medicine that will make you sleepy," he said to me.

"Do you watch *Garfield*?" I asked.

"Yes, I love lasagna," he replied.

"Me too," I said as I fell asleep in Mom's arms before I was taken to the operating room (OR). During the procedure, the surgeon, Dr. Hunter, reconstructed my mitral valve, the valve that lets blood flow from the left atrium to the left ventricle. He put in a plastic ring to restore the correct shape of the valve and reduce the regurgitation of blood. The ring had been used on only six other patients before me. He also ligated, or tied off, the abnormal, left coronary artery.

March 28, 1989

"Oh, Emily! You're waking up," a nurse said. "Emily, you're okay."

"I'm thirsty," I said hoarsely.

"Here you go," said the nurse, wetting a green sponge on the end of a white stick and placing it into my open mouth.

I eagerly sucked the cool, stale water off the sponge, which the nurse dipped into a Dixie cup to make it wet again.

"More," I begged.

"We have to be careful," the nurse said. "We don't want you to choke."

But I want more; I'm so thirsty. Looking at the side of my bed, I saw my IV pole with my Winnie the Pooh stuffed animal taped to the top.

The nurse kindly talked to me while checking my IV. "We taped your arm to the board so you don't see anything or touch it." Pale pink tape secured the gauze covering the IV.

Everyone says I'm so sensitive to everything. I'm glad the IV's covered. I gratefully looked back up at my bear and drifted back to sleep.

Two days after the surgery, I was moved from the Surgical Intensive Care Unit to the IMCU. I was in a room with other patients who had all kinds of procedures and I shared the television with a young girl next to me. The television hung from the ceiling at the foot of our beds in the middle of the space where the yellow curtain that separated us ended.

"What do you want to watch today?" I asked the girl.

"Let's watch cartoons."

We laughed at the jokes together. Soon after, I heard the cart coming down the hall before seeing the phlebotomist. The technician wheeled into the room with her brown box and glass vials with multicolored lids. She stopped at the foot of my bed and pulled out the tourniquet.

"NO!" I yelled, crying. "Not until my mom gets here!"

The technician tried to gently persuade me to calm down, but I only cried harder. I knew my tiny, uncooperative veins would cause problems.

"Do mine first," said my neighbor. "Her mom will be here soon."

A few hours later, a hospital volunteer said, "Time for arts and crafts! What will you do today, Emily? Yesterday you made that pretty bracelet of beads that spelled your name."

"Today, I'll paint a parrot."

"Oh! Lovely!" She wheeled me down the hall to the crafts area.

The next morning, a new phlebotomist, who did not know to wait for Mom, came to my bedside. I screamed and cried louder than ever before, trying to stop her and kicking my feet in the bed, making a real racket. My actions didn't set off any heart alarms and I got to demonstrate some of my newfound strength. From the elevator my mother heard me crying and hurried to my bedside, arriving just in time so that I didn't need to have the test without her.

The following day the nurse said, "You're doing so much better. We're going to move you into a private room with just one roommate. Also, your chest tubes aren't draining much at all anymore. You can get them out this evening."

I'll be glad to have these tubes gone. Although they are called chest tubes and drain the fluid around the lungs, the tubes come out of the skin above the belly button. There were three drainage tubes. *This will be okay. It's not a needle being put in, it's something being taken out.*

Later that evening a new nurse came into my room to remove the tubes.

"Lie on your side, and I'll pull the tubes out," the nurse said.

"Emily, we'll wait in the hall," Mom said, and she and Dad left.

I closed my eyes tightly, scared, but I did what I was told. I felt a strange intense tugging from deep inside. *My guts are going to spill out!* I began to cry, but the terrible feeling ended after a minute.

"Good job. You can sit up."

I opened my eyes and sat up, making sure my gown covered my stomach. My parents came back into the room and we learned about a new task.

"Emily will have to start using an incentive spirometer to make her lungs stronger."

The nurse handed me a clear plastic box with numbers on the front. I held the handle on one side and inhaled hard to raise the yellow ball to a measured height. *I'll do a bunch of short breaths. It will be over sooner.*

"Well, that's not where we want it to be, but we'll try again later," the nurse said to my parents.

After I brushed my teeth that night, the nurse brought the spirometer out again. "Let's give this another try, Emily. I know you can move the ball higher."

I hate this thing. I'm not doing it! I shook my head no, knowing Mom and Dad weren't there to reprimand me, and I refused to use it.

The next morning, the new nurse brought out the spirometer. "Time for morning breaths," she announced.

Taking several shallow breaths, I tried to get it over with as quickly as possible. *I'll fake it so they leave me alone.*

"Emily, can't you move the ball higher than that?" asked the nurse. I shook my head no. The nurse sighed and put the spirometer back on the table by my bedside. "Let's go for a walk."

I was tired and didn't want to walk. Just past the nurses' station, I said I needed to sit down. We went back to my room.

When the respiratory therapist came in, he instructed me to cough. I refused. Coughing hurt. "Let me see what you can do here," he said, handing me the spirometer. I took some shallow breaths and he recorded the numbers on my chart.

The doctor came to visit me a couple days later while my parents were in the room. "Emily has pneumonia," he told them. "She hasn't been walking, coughing, or using her spirometer enough. Now she has phlegm in her lungs. She'll have to stay here another week to recover."

April 1989

In a private hospital bathroom, Mom helped me disrobe. Gingerly getting into a warm soapy bathtub, I held onto Mom's arm. I played with the bubbles for a moment while Mom rolled up her sleeves. "It's time to wash the dissolvable stitches and tape from your chest," Mom said.

I looked down at my chest and saw clear, rigid plastic tape strips that were thicker than usual desk tape going horizontally down my upper body. The tape was yellow-brown from the solution used on my skin to sterilize it prior to the surgery. Mom handed me a large sponge and together we washed the tape and sticky goo off. *This isn't scary and it doesn't hurt. My scar's purple!*

Once it was visible, I saw a scar about eight inches long going down my chest with a raised portion at the bottom. There were also three purple spots on my stomach from the chest tubes. I said, "It's a snake with the three meals of breakfast, lunch, and dinner to eat."

The following day, April 12th, as I lay in the hospital bed, my phone rang. Mom handed me the phone.

"Hello?" I wasn't used to receiving calls in the hospital. I didn't want my friends to know about my heart condition, not wanting to be seen as different or weak, and I hadn't let them or my family visit me there.

"Emily, it's Grandma," she said with her strong New York accent. "I'm here with Sam and we're excited that you're coming home tonight! We're going to make you any kind of cookie you want."

"Peanut butter," I shouted, already dreaming of the sweet taste.

When I cautiously walked into the house, two and half weeks after I had left it, the air smelled sugary and nutty. I saw Grandma, with her always professionally set, pale-gray, ear-length hair, sitting by the oven. She came over and presented a tray of warm golden-brown cookies with crisscross fork indentations. "Here you go!"

I savored every sweet bite, feeling as though I was getting my well-deserved reward for what I had been through.

In late April, about a month after the surgery, I visited my first-grade class at school. They didn't know the specifics of why I was out, but they knew I'd been gone a long time and they missed me. As I slowly walked in, my classmates rushed toward me and enveloped me in hugs, telling me how glad they were to see me.

"Don't hug her too tight, Brendan," my teacher cautioned. "Be careful, her chest is delicate." It didn't hurt, I was so glad to see everyone.

My classmates gave me a pile of drawings and my teacher gave Mom books and assignments for me to catch up on at home. "She won't be able to come back to school until June, probably," Mom told my teacher quietly in the corner of the room. "She has to continue to rest and heal at home."

"Mrs. Neth, our classroom aide, will tutor her at your home and bring her assignments and anything else she misses," my teacher said.

Mom agreed with the plan, and said to me, "Emily, it's time to go home now."

I frowned and looked at my friend Katie. "Bye for now. I'll see you soon." She gave me a light hug and I waved goodbye to everyone as I left.

Mrs. Neth came to see me ten or fifteen times during the forty-five days I missed school. She was a tall woman with tanned skin and light brown-blonde curly hair. I noticed that she wore a diamond ring with the rock in the shape of an actual diamond, which stood out to me because it was similar to the diamond ring in one of my favorite movies, *Gentlemen Prefer Blondes*. She was the first person I ever knew to own an engagement ring in that shape.

We spent about six hours per week studying so that I could catch up with everything I had missed. Sitting together in the formal dining room, we spread out our weekly tasks across the big brown wooden table. Mrs. Neth brought me assignments and cards from my classmates. We made flashcards on note cards with stickers to help me learn about school subjects.

Most weeks we played my favorite non-school-related game together. Mrs. Neth had a wristwatch with a face surrounded by a ring that could change color. She'd ask me, "What color was my watch last week?"

I closed my eyes and conjured up an image of her watch and eagerly responded with whatever color I remembered. Whenever I guessed correctly, she would reward me with candy prizes like a box of Valentine's candy hearts. I'd line up my hearts in order of taste preference, saving the best for last. I looked forward to the game with its sweet rewards and never failed, thanks to my sharp observational skills. I was never great in school and didn't enjoy it; however, I liked learning with Mrs. Neth and playing our special games.

When I wasn't working on school assignments, I played with Sam. Sometimes we went on short walks to slowly rebuild my stamina.

About five weeks after the surgery, I had a checkup with my surgeon, Dr. Hunter. I found Dr. Hunter to be a large, intimidating man. His dark hair and beard made him seem larger than life, and the power he held over my fate made me feel nervous owing to the weight of his words. During my postoperative (postop) office visit, I sat on the exam table on top of the crinkly wax paper, and he gave me a small brown teddy bear with a red heart stitched on its chest. His gift disarmed me, and I relaxed.

In a booming voice he said, "You can run, swim, or go up the stairs as much as you feel like."

Elated, once the appointment was over, I grabbed Dad's hand and went to visit the staff from the floor where I stayed after my surgery.

"Look what I can do!" I said and ran halfway down the hall.

The nurses grinned and cheered me on.

After the surgery, I didn't have insomnia; but when I woke up early in the morning, I could not fall back to sleep (common after open-heart surgery). I left my room in the early hours ahead of sunrise and went to watch TV in the living room, to pass the time before my family woke up. I kept the volume low, flipping past *The Jetsons* and *The Pink Panther* to the paid programming channel. There I watched my favorite show, a St. Jude's fundraising program featuring children with cancer. Children in the hospital were documented going through medical tests and they were interviewed, discussing their illnesses.

A girl on the show had lost her hair, and she had a long-term IV and visible scars. She detailed her medical care and all of the treatment she had been through. It was riveting watching kids describe some of the tests and pain I also had experienced but couldn't talk about with anyone. I curled my hair around my finger and buttoned up my shirt to hide my scar when I heard Mom coming out and quickly changed the channel to a cartoon, still replaying the girl's words in my head.

Two months after surgery, in May, I had a checkup with my favorite doctor, Dr. Gold. My parents and I rode the elevator down to the bottom floor of the hospital and exited into a long hallway with low curved white ceilings and rust-colored floor tiles. We smelled the daily patient meals as we walked by the kitchens, hearing the pans clanging and passing by the racks full of hospital food trays with large silver covers waiting to be distributed in the hall.

On every occasion, Dr. Gold warmly welcomed me into his office, where I sat across from his desk in an area with two green child-sized mushroom-shaped stools and a table. I never sat on top of a large exam table, which made me feel much more relaxed and as if I were in a playroom, rather than at a medical office. He was a warm and caring man with a deep golden tan, kind blue eyes, and curly gray hair.

Dr. Gold blew warm air onto the diaphragm of the stethoscope before listening to my heart. He looked into my eyes and asked me sincerely but merrily, "Is this warm enough?" while tentatively placing it under my shirt on my chest waiting to hear my answer.

"Yep," I agreed, even if it was chilly. Dr. Gold never made me feel anxious, simply well cared for and special.

"You're healing beautifully. You can go back to school in the mornings for a few hours a day."

I smiled at my parents, knowing this was a good step.

With my new energy, I ran up and down hallways at home and around the neighborhood. At the end of May, I resumed swimming, an activity I loved to do both before and after surgery. In July, on a walk after dinner, I did some running and rode my bike pretty far. *I can't believe I did that. I'm so much better now.* Both activities were new for me to experience, and for my parents to see.

Years later, I once asked Mom how she knew I was thriving after the surgery. She said, "One night at dinner, you requested a second serving. You'd never done that before." It was a real sign I was getting better. As a result of my gaining weight, my ribs no longer protruded from my chest. My previously overworked heart was enlarged and had pushed my ribs out to make space and now they weren't as noticeable.

September 1989

After my lengthy absence from first grade and attending summer school, I returned for second grade. Special considerations were provided to me and I was placed in a classroom that combined first and second graders, helping me to catch up on the schooling I had missed. After school I ran across the street from the bus stop to my front door, excited to play with Sam. While we played, I said, "Aren't you happy I don't have to nap anymore when I get home and we can play together?"

"Yes, Emmy!" she said.

At the end of September, I decided to ride my bike on a raw, autumn New England day. Overcome with an unusual burst of confidence, I wanted to show off for Grandma to demonstrate I could now ride my bike around the neighborhood and raced down a steep hill. Even though I was warned the roads were slick, I proceeded on my bike and paid the price. My bike wheels slipped on the wet leaves from rain earlier in the week. I heard screeching tires and blood rushing to my ears as I fell at the bottom of the hill onto my chin. The entire neighborhood could hear me howling in tears as Grandma walked me home. When we entered the house Mom sighed. "I don't remember you wearing a red shirt ..."

She quickly handed me washcloths to soak up the blood coming from my chin. Grandma stayed at home with Sam, while Mom and I made the familiar drive into the city to MGH to be where all my specialists were in case my heart reacted to this injury. I clutched onto the soaked towels and we drove in silence, hearing only the other cars whizzing by on the highway and my soft sniffles. In the ER, the doctors could see the white bone of my chin when I removed the washcloths I had been tightly clinging to, terrified to remove them for fear of receiving stitches. In the end, I was left with a scar and yellow and white fuzzy stickers of bears the nurse gave me when the black scratchy stitches, hard like animal whiskers, were removed. Those bears were the envy of all my friends in school.

That was the same year I finally started growing at an average rate. My stamina was improving and I could manage to walk from house to house trick-or-treating for two hours, instead of being driven as I had been previously. I painted my face green and wore a black witch's hat with a sparkly silver star and a black dress, victoriously heaping up the candy.

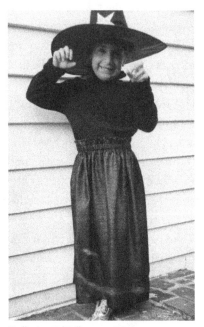

Emily, Age 7 (Halloween, 1989)

Learning to Cope with Being Different

"How are you feeling, Emily?" asked my therapist, whom I saw before and after surgery. He sat on his couch across from me in his office, which was in his house rather than in a medical building. We played games at our sessions and talked throughout. The most frequent game we played was *Sorry!* Players try to get their pieces from start to home on the board and along the way you can hit pieces to send them back to the starting line. Angrily hitting the therapist's pieces with my navy-blue token allowed me to take out my aggression.

"Are you mad?" he asked. "It's normal to be mad."

I wouldn't meet his eyes. Instead, I rolled the little blue man across the table.

It's not fair. Other kids don't have scars.

"You know you can tell me how it feels."

You can't understand. I pushed the dice over to him and refused to talk about certain feelings.

Salt

I sat down in the elementary school lunchroom opening my lunch bag to find another tuna fish sandwich, which I slowly ate. Mom made me a sandwich every day, and I never got to buy school lunch. I liked Mom's cooking, but I was envious of the kids having pizza. Prior to the surgery, I was in congestive heart failure from infancy to age six (my heart wasn't failing, it just wasn't efficient). I couldn't have school-made pizza since I couldn't have much salt, if any, because salt can make liquid retention worse for congestive heart failure. Even though I was no longer in failure, I had to limit salt and fluids as a precaution.

At a friend's home when I was in second grade, several friends and I sat at her long dining room table to celebrate her birthday. Colorful streamers filled the room with balloons bouncing on the ceiling as the festive lunch was served. The meal included potato chips. Unbeknownst to me, Mom had dropped me off in the morning along with salt-free potato chips for me to eat; I had no idea and thought I was eating what everyone else was.

Coping with Restrictions on Physical Activities

All the physical activities I enjoyed I did with my family, never with peers. While my classmates went to gym class, I worked in the main administrative office. As my schoolmates ran outside to play, I walked to the office and cheerily asked the administrative staff, "What am I doing today?" They assigned me tasks like organizing the supply cabinet next to the copy machine, which had flickering lights as it spit out copies. I stayed busy until gym class was over. I wasn't envious of my friends, since I enjoyed organizing and stuffing envelopes with class assignments for the following year. My friends begged me to tell them which teacher they would have next year, but I kept my mouth shut.

At recess, I often played by myself quietly, sitting in the wooden castle structure and making up stories. Occasionally, I'd watch my classmates play soccer. Since I was invisible to my classmates when it came to sports, I was never offered another task like scorekeeping. I sat on the sidelines, pulling up grass stems and hiding my loneliness about being left out. Over time, I learned how to control my reactions to being excluded. I knew not to ask to try physical things, since they were off-limits.

After a while, the teachers started letting me attend gym class. My parents had told me not to share medical information unless it pertained to physical activities. Gym class required me to expose the truth. "What can't you do?" was a question commonly asked by strangers, teachers, and friends when my condition was revealed.

I responded with the mantra I learned to recite about my restrictions and all the activities I could *not* do since I was never told what I *could* do or try outside of my normal, safe routine, "No weight lifting, no endurance activities, and no joining a sports team."

"Oh, my. Can you play tag?"

I shrugged because I probably had never tried to do it before. "I guess I could try a little," I'd venture, looking around warily for teachers or parents who might stop me if they saw what I was doing. Neither the doctors nor I could precisely define the boundaries. After running a short distance, I always knew when to stop if it was too much and I required a rest. If I did try to push myself a little and became out of breath, I didn't feel like I had done any damage to my heart, but I couldn't be sure, so I remained cautious. I was never scared by my heart, only scared of making the doctors and my family mad.

Family Accommodations

My family and I went on many vacations together when I was younger. We did not go on adventure vacations, physically active trips, or to places at high altitude. When I was eight, we went to the Southwest in the United States. I was incapable of doing much hiking, so neither could my family. "Emily, Dad and Sam are going to go ahead and see some of the rocks up that hill."

I watched them recede into the distance in the hot sun and sat under a tree with Mom. I kept myself busy playing in the sand, oblivious to what I was missing.

When they returned, I asked, "What'd you see?"

Sam replied, "Some orange rocks and a lizard. Dad took a picture for you." *I'm glad Sam didn't forget about me and Dad took a photo, but I'm still jealous.*

Follow-Up Appointments

After the first surgery, I went to the doctor for check-ups only once every six months. Constant anxiety over cardiac emergencies slowly slipped away. Mom and I sat in hospital waiting rooms, awaiting tests or medical appointments. We browsed the magazine selection in front of us. *American Association of Retired Persons, Reader's Digest,* and *Better Homes and Gardens* stared back at us. I looked at all of the gray-haired patients around me, frustrated that none of the reading choices interested me. Curious stares were returned from people wondering what I was doing in the waiting room with them.

Sometimes the patients and I spoke. "What are you, such a young girl, doing here? You can't have a heart condition."

"I do, and I've had it since I was born," I self-consciously replied.

Shocked, the patients would say they had just become ill themselves and asked me questions about tests and experiences I had gone through that they were about to experience for the first time. *I wish you had what I have. It's always only me. No one's ever my age. I wonder if I'll ever meet anyone with my condition.*

Once a year, there was a picnic for cardiac patients and their families at Boston Children's Hospital. My family and I attended the picnic for three years, from right before I turned six until I was eight years old.

On a bright, sunny summer day at my last picnic, I ran off into the grass with a young girl. We looked at stickers together and she asked, "Do you have a heart problem?"

"Yes, do you?"

"No, my brother does."

We went back to playing and didn't talk about hearts anymore.

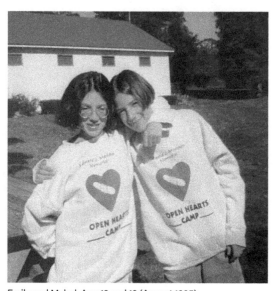
Emily and Mabel, Age 12 and 13 (August 1995)

Open Hearts Camp

At ten years old, in the summer between fourth and fifth grade, I began attending the Edward J. Madden Open Hearts Camp (OHC) in Great Barrington, Massachusetts. The camp is tailored to meet the needs of children who have experienced open-heart surgery. The year before I attended, my parents and I visited on a day trip, to learn what OHC offered. We went on a tour with the camp director, who gave us a short history: "In 1961, one of the first open-heart surgery patients created this camp. He wanted cardiac children to have a place to enjoy nature and sports together, without the pressure of keeping up with noncardiac kids. A place where they were not pushed beyond their limits and were not ashamed to slow down if they needed to."[6] This man, Edward Madden, turned his own home into a haven for children to feel welcome and safe.

My parents smiled and I could tell they thought this would be an excellent experience for me. *I might fit in here! I can't believe there's so many people like me that all the beds are filled.*

Camp was located in the Berkshires, a hilly region in Western Massachusetts. Upon arrival in Great Barrington every summer, the car windows were filled with sights of rolling green hills. As I lowered the windows, the fresh scent of grass filled my nostrils, and I heard the silence of the countryside, occasionally interrupted by the buzzing of insects and cars passing by. The camp was situated on a rural road, marked by a white picket fence. Every August when I attended camp, I felt giddy anticipation as the fence came into view from a mile away. It was a welcoming beacon that signaled my return for four years.

The large white buildings at camp were the main house where we ate, the recreation (rec) room, and two dorms, one for girls and one for boys. Each dorm had twenty beds separated on two sides. Both sides of the dorm had about seven campers and there were single beds with a dresser for each person and a shared bathroom. The groups were designed to be small to ensure kids got the attention they needed, but it also encouraged a familial feeling between the staff and campers. There was one camp counselor per dorm side, a camp director, a nurse, and assistants who prepared our food and did our laundry. Campers were expected to dress for dinner and make their beds. It was a home away from home.

Where's Your Scar?

Once the camp session began, I quickly made friends and settled in, finally feeling the sense of community I had longed for. As friendships grew, the loneliness and isolation I experienced from a young age vanished. For two weeks out of the year I got to be a normal kid.

Campers rarely talked about their conditions, but everyone had been through something, even if we didn't know or understand the details of our medical histories. The words and experiences of EKG and echo were familiar, but I wasn't aware of the other conditions the children had; I understood only that they weren't mine. Some people had gone through their medical experiences as babies and remembered nothing. Although it was not as common, others like me were older when they were operated on. Some of us, including me, stood in line at the nurse's office after breakfast to take daily medication. I might have asked friends why they didn't take medication, but it wasn't a big deal. Someone was always in line with me, unlike in elementary school where I waited alone for my daily medication at the nurse's office.

On my first morning at camp, I woke up early as I normally did at home. I noticed another camper was also awake. *Friends at home during sleepovers are never up this early like me.*

I got up from my creaking bed and met her on the floor in between our beds.

"What's your doll's name?" I whispered.

"Ellie. What's yours?"

My new camper friend and I played together, waiting for the others to wake up. It was nice to have a connection already with someone in a different way than my friends at home.

One of my first camp counselors was a past camper.

"You had surgery, too?" I asked her. *Wow. Someone's older than me. Most kids don't grow up. She's so pretty.*

"Yes, when I was a kid. Now I'm going to become a heart surgeon."

"Tell me about college. What's it like?" I eagerly waited for her answers.

I wrote home to my family, "We had 'nottles' [noodles] for lunch." Another day at lunch, I ate peanut butter and Fluff for the first time. The marshmallow gooeyness was intoxicating, and I lunged at the jar on the table whenever I had the chance to coat my sandwiches with it. In one letter during my first year at camp, I let my parents know "Joe fell on a stick and went to the hospital and got three stitches." My tooth fell out after I arrived my first year, I scraped my finger with a fishing hook my third year, and during my last year I had my first period. No one made a big deal about minor body events because we all knew what it was like to experience the giant stuff.

My first summer, when we went to the swimming pool, I tightly wrapped my black and rainbow square towel around my body, being sure to cover my chest. After claiming a lounge chair, I saw the returning campers proudly shed their towels and run around without any self-consciousness about their appearance. I looked around, trying not to stare, and saw that kids who had experienced more than one surgery had thicker or darker scars than mine; those who had surgery when they were babies had barely visible scars. Some campers even had scars near their lungs on their back, something I'd never seen previously. I quickly got used to this new feeling of freedom, dropped my towel on the chair, and happily played in the water, never thinking about anything other than finding my Marco Polo partner.

Once, a staff member's child who was heart healthy went swimming with us, and several campers questioned where her scar was. She was the odd one out, for not having a scar. We all enjoyed feeling like our scarred bodies fit in with the group and we appreciated playing together like typical children.

When I grew cold in the pool, my lips turned purple. Normally I was teased about this by friends at home as I shivered, cold and embarrassed. At camp, almost everyone else in the pool had purple and blue lips, too, our own special punk lipstick that couldn't be replicated by any cosmetics company. Around the same time, we all got out of the pool to warm up, lying on our lounge chairs baking in the sun together.

Participating at Camp

At camp, I thrived. It was one of the only places where there was no need to hide anything from anyone. Everyone was "the heart kid." The staff knew how to cater to all of us and handle our varied limitations. No one was excluded.

Currently, most cardiologists encourage children to try to do more and are told by their families that they can do anything. This wasn't the case for me and for many of my peers. At camp, I wasn't on the sidelines for any activities, which was new to me.

"Emily, try to hit the softball, then run at your own pace to the base," the counselor told me.

"They'll be mad if I'm slow," I replied.

"No, we won't! We're all slow!" one of the seasoned campers shouted.

"Sure, I'll try." I could exert myself somewhat, still adhering to my restrictions, given leeway and understanding based on needs.

We played softball, kickball, and kick-the-can, and practiced archery. We hiked and climbed large rocks, fished in a stream, and took care of pet salamanders, my favorite activity. I was sometimes at the front of the group on hikes, sometimes at the back. At times, my rest breaks could be longer or shorter than what the other campers needed. In one letter I wrote home, I proudly stated, "We went bowling and I was the only one who got a strike!" When it rained, we played board games, pool, and air hockey in the rec room, or watched movies. As the undisputed air-hockey champion during all of my years at camp, I couldn't be beat. I boasted in a letter to my family, "I played air hockey and I won by a lot of points every time!" I could be myself without being self-conscious about my abilities, and most important of all, I never felt judged.

A New Best Friend Forever

At camp I met my lifelong best friend: my co-camper, Mabel. My first week at camp during my first year, I immediately noticed outspoken, outgoing, and confident Mabel. At once, I was drawn to this short, pale camper with black hair, boldly wearing green glasses. She had a constant tiny line of blue on her bottom pink lip, the single outward sign she had a cardiac condition other than her scars. She was tough even though she was a year younger than me and much louder, with a strong New York accent at times.

When we set up our beds and space around them, Mabel and I both hung up posters of teen heartthrobs from magazines. We liked the same television stars and books and became inseparable, bonding over our common interests. Mabel was always the center of attention. To us campers she seemed sophisticated, knowing everything about pop culture, boys, and fashion. All the girls tried to become her best friend, but I won the prized spot. We enjoyed writing together during our rest periods and made up stories about the lives we dreamed of having when we grew up. Together we played the card game Spit and we read a lot. We shared tapes that we listened to on our Walkmans and sang loudly to songs together on the swings in the summer sun. A favorite was "Finally" by CeCe Peniston. I wrote to my parents, "Me and Mabel are having a lot of fun, so you won't be getting as many letters."

One day at camp we went into town to shop. Mabel and I hurried off away from the group to do our own thing in Walmart.

"Look at these frogs," Mabel said as she came across a stuffed animal pile. We examined them closely together and chose a pair. Mabel took the lead saying, "I'll name my red frog Herb."

"Then mine is Herby," I said about my yellow frog, always trying to keep up with her.

When we got back to camp we settled in and during our rest period that day, I said, "I'm going to do surgery on Herby."

"What do you mean, is he sick?" Mabel said, concerned.

"No," I laughed. "I'm removing his tag! Not everything is about hearts!"

When Mabel and I went on hikes in the woods, I usually was ahead of her going up the hills. Not having the same heart condition, we had different levels of physical ability. She was often at the back of the pack, but we never discussed our separation and naturally met at the end of the activity. Sometimes I slowed my pace to walk with her and she'd do the same for me when I was at the rear. It was okay if we didn't do the whole hike together and it didn't matter who got there first. Sometimes one of us needed a break and didn't want to make a fuss about it. We didn't need to explain things to each other like we did with other kids, making our friendship effortless. Our bond went beyond liking the same things; it was a deep, empathetic understanding. Every night, we fell asleep holding hands, talking about our day.

An activity during the camp session was visiting a local peacock farm. We rode in the camp van, over the state line into New York, where Mabel was from. As we picked up as many feathers as we could find in rainbows of greens, blues, and even white, Mabel proudly pointed out, "I'm home and you're not!" This was about as competitive as we ever got. Hearing the loud screeching of the peacocks as they defended their home was exciting and a tad like proud Mabel.

Although "camp" might conjure up rustic images, this camp also had formal elements. We had to wear dresses to dinner every night. Mabel and I helped each other pick out our outfits and do our hair listening to pop music as we got ready. Dinner was served promptly at six every night and whichever camper was ready first for dinner, standing outside of the dining hall, got to ring the bell to inform the other campers it was dinner time. Sitting on the bed watching Mabel do her hair, long after mine was done, I'd say, "Come on, hurry up, I want to ring the bell!"

"I'm trying," she'd laugh and say, "Go without me." Unlike on our hikes, in this situation I could never leave my best friend and waited on the edge of the bed.

On the last night of camp, there was a dance. We wore dresses we had not worn to dinner and danced in the rec room with our dates and friends. Throughout the two weeks leading up to the dance, we'd try to figure out which boy should take us to the dance. During hikes, Mabel and I held hands with different boys to get to know them better and see if we were a match. Sweaty palms and nerves often got in my way, but almost immediately, Mabel found her Mr. Right. There was no question about who would greet her at the door and take her to the dance.

Before we left our dorm, Mabel rushed to get ready and was a bit ahead of schedule. She had made the time to do my makeup for the dance. Since she has an older sister, she knew much more about fashion and makeup than I did. She made me look beautiful with bright pink lipstick and blue eyeshadow to match my blue dress. We danced the night away with each other rather than our dates for some songs and I played air hockey in the rec room while she danced with Mr. Right.

The best part of the night was when we returned to our dorm after the dance, when we ate the candy our parents had packed for us prior to leaving home. It was like Halloween, with all the girls sitting on the floor, trading candy pieces and enjoying the treats that had been forbidden until the last night as our special end-of-summer treat. We exchanged addresses so we could write to each other once we returned home. The next day, our parents came to pick us up and we performed a talent show for them. Mabel and I always chose to lip-sync songs and dance together. One year we performed "Summer Nights" from *Grease*. I wore a dress I had worn to dinner and borrowed a white sweater to play Sandy, while Mabel wore a slick leather jacket to act as Danny. We used the camp picnic table for Sandy's part and the porch of the dorm as the location for Danny's solo, like in the movie. The crowd loved it, and it was a huge hit.

Staying in Touch

Throughout the year between summers, Mabel and I sent each other letters and spoke once a week on the phone. In July 1994, just before I turned twelve, I called Mabel to tell her about my family vacation.

"We went to see Mt. St. Helens and something crazy happened."

"What? Did you fall off the mountain?" Mabel asked.

I laughed, "No, I fell asleep on the car ride up. I couldn't keep my eyes open the higher we went. Sam tried to poke me to keep me awake but I couldn't wake up, so they drove back down."

"Oh my gosh. Do you think your heart made you tired?"

"Yeah, I guess. The doctors and my parents didn't know that would happen. Does it happen to you?"

"No, not that I've noticed."

"My family missed seeing stuff. I wish they'd gone ahead without me so they wouldn't have to miss things." I sighed.

"I know, me too. It's hard."

"My mom's calling. I have to get off the phone, but I'll see you on Instant Messenger after school. We can plan our winter and summer visits soon, too."

"You bet," Mabel replied and we hung up.

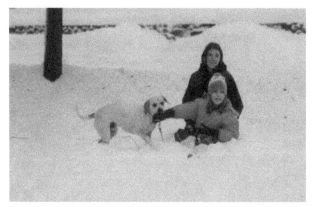

Emily, Age 13, Sam, Age 8, and Benny on a Snow Day (December 1995)

Relationships with Doctors

It was always exhilarating to wake up to the sound of the town's chime signifying a snow day. I kicked my blankets off and hurried to get ready for the day, relishing the freedom from middle school. Dressed in my parka, snow pants, and warm hat I rushed outside to the pristine white yard. Squinting in the light, I surveyed the area and plopped down in a fluffy patch of white to make snow angels and lick the tasty, untouched snow. The cold snowflakes danced on my eyelashes and cheeks while I heard my family shoveling the driveway. Their scraping shovels and sounds of exertion made me envious.

Lifting heavy snow can be too strenuous and can put a sudden strain on the heart. Hearing shovels chopping ice in a methodical rhythm in the driveway, I occasionally kicked the snow, trying secretly to help out. *I'm always getting good news from the doctor. I can try some of this,* I thought as I lifted a block of ice, out of my parents' line of vision. When my parents saw me, though, they told me to stop. Not stubborn enough to fight them, I let it go. I quit trying to join in, as I did with so many other things in life. I ran off to another part of the yard to make snowmen and throw snowballs at Sam.

Dr. Gold's Retirement

At my winter appointment when I was twelve, I went to see my pediatric cardiologist, Dr. Gold. Since he was one of the few doctors I liked and looked forward to seeing, I brought him a gift. "I made you this ceramic heart in pottery class," I told him.

"Thank you, Emily. That's so kind of you, especially because I have to tell you I'll no longer be your doctor."

I swallowed my tears and looked at Mom, wondering if she'd changed my doctor without telling me.

"I'm retiring," he said, "so this will be our last appointment together." He gave me a big hug and we left his basement office for the last time.

On the drive home, I traced the outline of my new heart pin that said, "Hands Off." Mom bought it for me in the hospital gift shop trying to console me. I asked her through tears, "What will I do now?"

"He's taken the best care of you anyone could, but your new doctor will care for you, too," she said.

I doubt it. I rolled my eyes and looked out the window imagining all the tests I'd seen on television that a new doctor might prescribe, afraid for my next appointment. When I got home, I signed on to Instant Messenger to talk to Mabel.

"Dr. Gold's leaving. I don't know what I'm going to do. This new person's probably awful."

"I've had my doctor forever. He's not going anywhere."

"It's not fair," I typed angrily.

Dr. Smith

I began seeing Dr. Smith, an adult congenital heart disease cardiologist. Even though he had helped care for me since I was an infant and had always been involved in my care, I had no memory of him.

Dr. Smith's office was not in the main hospital building. I walked through a parking lot in a residential apartment complex near the hospital and entered a medical building. On the first floor, I walked into a large room with mammoth revolving filing shelves that reached from the floor to the ceiling with patient records. Sitting in a stiff, black wooden chair I glanced around the room at the drawings of golden retrievers on the walls. I waited to be called for an EKG. *My file is so thick compared to the others on the shelves.*

After the test was completed by a technician, I returned to the waiting room. Dr. Smith was a busy man, with many patients. As an expert on adult congenital heart disease, he was in demand and his workload was increasing exponentially. *How much longer do I have to wait? It's been hours already. I guess he's answering lots of questions today.* Silently, patients of all ages and I looked at each other or read magazines, as tension filled the air.

Eventually, I'd hear Dr. Smith's office door open, and he came out in his usual suit and tie. He approached the shelf on his administrative assistant's desk where files for that day's patients were piled high. My heart pounded and my palms were sweaty as he picked up the top folder and, in a booming voice, looked to his left and called out, "Emily Anne!"

That's not my middle name, I growled in my head, but I stood up smiling and walked over to him. He enveloped me warmly in a hug, and I pretended to genuinely hug him back (although I felt terror and anger). He put his arm around me and pushed me along into his office by the small of my back.

Once inside, he sat behind a bulky, carved wooden desk. I looked under the glass top and saw hundreds of photos of patients he had cared for throughout the years. The white walls of this bright sunny room were lined with photographs of destinations he had visited and famous patients he had treated. The room was clean and orderly, but it lacked the warmth of Dr. Gold's office.

Interrupted by the phone, he listened and said, "Yes, take that medicine. I'll be at the hospital in a few hours." His importance filled the room.

I listened to whatever confidential details I could glean from the conversation as I waited my turn. *It's probably someone calling for his advice from some distant country.* He was extremely reliable, always reachable by phone or email, but not always approachable; he was more business-like than the warm and fuzzy Dr. Gold.

Sitting meekly in front of this man, with his thinning brown hair parted to the side, I rarely made eye contact with him and slouched in my chair. He read my EKG results, reciting my condition for the medical students in the room. Dr. Smith took great interest in teaching (he eventually taught over five hundred cardiologists and internists) and always had several students in his office. After his speech, he started his barrage of questions for me. He read from a white form that he filled out at every visit, "Do you drink, do you smoke, are you taking your medications?"

I mumbled my answers and felt invisible. He didn't look up to see how I was reacting to his questions while I squirmed in the chair. Once the questions were over, it was time to listen to my heart. *I can't stand being on display like this. The students are lining up to examine me like I'm a museum exhibit.*

I shuffled to the back of his office and sat on the exam table. Dr. Smith listened to my heart and said, "Deep breath, in and out."

Inhaling and exhaling, sometimes I didn't put my full effort into it, depending on how irritated I felt. Dr. Smith moved his stethoscope around my chest, lungs, and back, intently listening, repeating the types of breaths he needed me to make. The cold steel bell provided some comfort since I'd done this for so many years and it never hurt me.

After listening to my heart and lungs, Dr. Smith explained to the students what to listen for. I smiled my fake smile as I was poked and prodded like a rare medical specimen. While the students examined my body, Dr. Smith spoke into his recorder at his desk, reciting my medical details and findings.

When Dr. Smith explained things to the medical students, I'd listen to try to figure things out about myself I didn't know. *I still don't know what he's talking about.* I lay still for more student exams. *He thinks I can understand the heart model on his desk, but I've got no clue. He's never explained it. I wish he'd draw a diagram and describe all this to me so what he's saying would make sense to me.* After listening to my heart and reciting what they heard to Dr. Smith, the students pinched my ankles, checking for swelling to make sure I wasn't in heart failure, and they took my blood pressure.

They never took the time to get to know me or ask me anything personal, merely responding to Dr. Smith's orders like worker bees who might have been afraid of him, too.

I'm too scared to ask him anything. I didn't want to waste his time on questions I thought he might consider trivial. *I guess I'm fine, he always says there's nothing to worry about. I don't need to make any decisions about tests, so I'll be quiet.*

With the exam completed, I slowly walked back to the chair in front of Dr. Smith's desk.

"You sound great."

I sighed inwardly. *Phew, but now what new thing will he prescribe?*

"I'm starting you on a new medication. It'll keep your blood pressure stable. Your heart will do less work, which will benefit you for longevity." I grinned my immense smile—my armor from anger and fear—and stayed silently furious as I sat across from him, nodding in agreement. *Mom and Dad say there's no one better than him. I have to do whatever he says.*

Dr. Smith continued to take notes as I stared at the floor. *I wonder if he'll bring up my last test and explain the results when he's done? Probably not, he only calls to tell me when something's wrong or I need another test. I hope I don't need an IV or have to do something showing everyone I'm sick.* Everything Dr. Smith did to treat me and keep my heart healthy for the future was working, I simply didn't know why. The lack of explanation and communication about tests made it hard to be thankful for Dr. Smith and all that he did for me.

"You need a Holter monitor, a portable device to measure and record your heartbeats like an EKG for the next twenty-four hours," he said.

"Why do I need one?" I tried to bravely ask. "I feel fine."

"Insurance," was a common answer I couldn't understand at the time.

I left Dr. Smith's office and went to the EKG room to be hooked up to the device. The EKG leads on my chest were attached to a portable cassette tape that recorded all of my heartbeats. The cassette's wheels made an electronic whirring noise, which was easy to hear in moments of silence. The tape was encased in a red box, the width of about two cassette tapes, which the technician attached to the top rim of my pants in a black pouch.

I'm so glad I wore my baggy shirt today with a high neck. I hope no one sees this. Uh oh. My stomach often got upset when leaving Dr. Smith's office.

After I returned home, free from school, the Holter monitor technician's voice echoed in my head, "*Live normally. Try to exercise a small amount and press the button if you feel anything irregular.*" Sometimes I lay like a lump on the couch in anger watching TV, barely moving, listening to the whirring of the tape. Other times, I would make an effort to record some exercise by walking my dog, Benny. Together we ran a little or walked briskly up and down hills to try to show how my heart reacted. At night, I slept with the monitor next to me, careful not to turn onto it or disconnect a lead.

The following morning, I stared at the clock in the bathroom, waiting for the minute to change to the twenty-four-hour mark when I could tear the EKG leads off. Hurriedly, I removed them and unclipped the tape from the top of my pants. I wrapped the machine in the return package to mail to Dr. Smith and put it in the hall for Mom to take to the post office. I then enjoyed a long shower, which was forbidden when wearing the machine, and washed all the sticky goo and memories away.

Spice Girls

In the summer of 1996, when I was fourteen, I spent the weekend at Mabel's home on Long Island. We went for a walk in her neighborhood and sat together on the grass. She said, "Have you heard of the Spice Girls?" She turned on her portable boom box that we brought to the park, and tuned to the radio station, Z100, to wait to hear their song. When the Spice Girls song "Wannabe" came on, I was in awe. *There'll never be a better song than this. Mabel knows me better than anyone else in the world.* When I got home Sunday, I called the local radio station, KISS 108, repeatedly to request the song. Finally, after what felt like hours of waiting, they played it. I screamed for Sam to come into the room and turned it up to full volume. I danced in circles around Benny, who was jumping onto my leg dancing with me while I held his paws, with Sam and Mom laughing, watching me.

A year later, in high school, I took a step-aerobics class and tried to dance to the new Spice Girls song. The teacher said, "Everyone, step up on the platform and then down again." To me she said loudly over the music, "Not you, Emily. You can't do that. Step to the side of the platform."

I swallowed my frustration and embarrassment as my cheeks turned red and did the same steps on the floor next to the green and purple platform, with no change in elevation. *I think I can do this, but I don't want to get into trouble.* After school, standing in the street, I stepped up on the curb and then back down again. *I don't get why I can't do this in class. I feel all right and my breathing's normal. This is so unfair. What's she going to do to me if I try in class? Kick me out?*

My school system had never had any students with a health condition like mine, but five years after I started attending school, they had another student that did.

"Emily, there's a boy in my class with a heart condition, too," Sam said. She was still in elementary school.

"I know his mother from our support group that we went to when you were younger," Mom chipped in. "He doesn't have what you have."

"He comes to gym class with me and plays with us," Sam said as I sat hiding my envy.

Junior year in high school, the gym teacher told my class to run at our own pace on the indoor track. "Except you, Emily. You're not doing it." I went home in tears.

"They let everyone participate except me," I cried to Mom. "It was at our own pace. I don't understand why I couldn't do it too."

"You could have. That's not acceptable," she said and called the school to speak to the teacher. I overheard her end of the conversation.

"No, that's not what I told the school nurse. She can participate at her own pace. She knows when to rest and won't push herself. You should've let her join in. It's not right that you embarrassed her like that," Mom said.

The following day at school, I walked up to the teacher and said, "You're going to have to get used to people with heart conditions as many of us are now surviving."

Volunteering at a Hospital

When I was sixteen, I started volunteering at Lahey Hospital and Medical Center. I worked on a patient floor and in Human Resources (HR).

One summer day, it was my job to refill the water pitchers in patient rooms. In one older man's room, I heard a nurse tell him he needed to have an EKG. When the nurse left he turned to me, whispering, "I'm so nervous. I've never had any tests on my heart."

"Well, you have the right volunteer," I laughed. "I've had open-heart surgery and a lifetime of tests."

"Really?" he said, wide-eyed.

"I can tell you all about it. There's no need to be afraid. They'll place twelve stickers on you, two on your ankles, two on your upper arms near your shoulders, five on the left side of your chest following your rib line, and two on your chest under your collarbone. The stickers don't hurt when they go on. They're a little cold from the goo they sometimes have on the underside. After the test is done, I like to peel them off myself so I can do it slowly so it hurts less, but sometimes the technician takes them off fast and then your skin gets red but it doesn't really hurt more than a few seconds. That's maybe the worst part, but it's nothing." I pointed to the white machine that was already in the room. "This box thing will print out a pink piece of paper with the reading from your heart. There'll be black lines in a squiggle showing your heart rhythm, and they give that to the doctor."

"I'm much less anxious now. Will you be there for the EKG?"

"Yes, of course. I can hold your hand and I'll even put the stickers on you."

I gently put the stickers on him and stayed in the room after the test to make sure the patient felt heard and taken care of.

Not all of my volunteer duties were so pleasant. A year later, while I was pouring water into a patient's cup, he suddenly started bleeding from his hand where his IV was placed. "I'm bleeding!" the patient shrieked. I looked over and saw his crisp white sheets turning red around his hand. *This isn't so bad, it's just a little bit.* The small spot started to grow. *I wish I knew how to help. I have to get someone! I don't like this.* I went out into the hall and found a nurse to help him.

At the end of August 2000, before leaving for college, I completed my two-year volunteer job at the hospital. There was a special ceremony to thank the volunteers, and we received commemorative plaques.

"I had such a great time here. I'll miss it," I told Mary, the Volunteer Coordinator.

"We'll miss you! You were here more hours than anyone else," she said.

"I enjoyed my time on the patient floors, but nursing shouldn't be my career. Unexpected blood, mine or a patient's, isn't for me." *Neither is being around doctors when it's not required.* I handed in my name badge and took my plaque home to show my family.

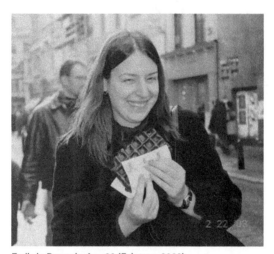

Emily in Brussels, Age 20 (February 2003)

Don't Waste a Second

When I returned home from college, I saw Dr. Smith on my own, without my parents, at my routine appointments with no other doctors in the room. *We're alone. It's so quiet. The phone's not ringing as much.*

"This year," he said, "I'm going to have you do a stress test during your winter break. You'll run on a treadmill for as long as you can and after, the technicians will inject you with a dye. Then you'll have an MRI, which will scan the dye and create a model of what's going on inside."

"Sure." I nodded. *Damn, an IV.*

"I know you're not happy about the IV, but I care for you, you're special to me. You were one of the most complicated patients. I lost more sleep and got more gray hairs from you and still do! I'm your mother hen, and I must take the best care of you that's possible."

It seems like he cares more now, maybe because no one's observing us. I left the appointment without an upset stomach for the first time.

At our summer appointment, prior to my turning twenty in 2002, Dr. Smith told me he was ramping down his appointments with patients.

"I'm transitioning your care over to Dr. Anderson. She's the new cardiologist in my practice. You met her last winter. I'll still be involved but she'll be the lead physician. Sometimes you'll only see her."

He's known me since I was baby. No one will ever know my heart better than him. I felt a panic similar to when Dr. Gold left. *I know he's trained the doctors, but they don't have as much experience.* I bit my cheek to keep from crying in front of him. *I hope I can still reach him easily.* "Okay, I guess," I said. "This year, for junior year, I want to study abroad in London for both semesters."

"Wow! What an opportunity. London's great. My stepdaughter lives there. You're going to have an amazing time. Your parents agreed?"

"Yep."

"I do, too. I know you can take care of yourself." He scribbled on a Post-it a list of his doctor friends I could contact if I had any problems. "Bring a year's supply of medicine. Stick to your usual restrictions and get your flu shot as always in the fall. Have fun!" he said.

Year Abroad in London

When I lived abroad, I went by a motto I made for myself, "Don't waste a second." Even if I had a cold or didn't feel motivated, I took advantage of every opportunity that came my way and made a point to go out into the city every day. The classroom building and dorm were attached, and my single room was on the second floor. *My first time having to take stairs to get to my room. I hope I'm able to do this every day.* I made friends with a group from my college in New Hampshire. We ate together in the dining hall and watched movies together in the evenings. Most of us didn't have friends outside of the school, with only each other to hang out with. The first week of classes, we met up in the television lounge. We took our calendars and class syllabi out. "I'm free the first and second weekend of next month. What about you?" my friend Jeff asked.

We compared the times we had free that overlapped and circled weekends we could spend together.

"Let's go to Amsterdam," Kate said. "I want to get a tattoo in Canterbury, too, when we go next week for class. Who's coming with me?"

With no classes on Fridays, we had a plan to spend at least one weekend together away from London almost every month of the fall semester.

We took the ferry to Amsterdam and toured the Heineken beer factory. Another weekend, my two friends, both named Mike, and I went to Wales. In pubs, I tried nachos that had an orange seasoning on them like paprika, not found at home.

I took classes that involved outings to the theater, where I saw several shows and met many actors afterward. At one theater performance, I met Colin Firth. I strode up to him bravely. *Don't be a chicken, talk to him, he's a person too.* "Hi, I'm Emily and I'd love to get a photo with you." *The one thing I'm brave at.*

"Hi! Let me get my agent to do it," he said and put his arm around me in a photo as I beamed.

For class credit, I traveled around England to see stately homes and castles. On a weekend trip to a large castle in the country, there were many stairs. "I'll sit out on this part," I told my teacher. "I'll meet you in the garden." I wandered around the ground floor of the castle and found a room with jewelry. The sparkles kept me busy and I met up with my class later.

"They shined so brightly and were so old," I told my friend on the bus ride home.

"I wish I'd seen that. All I saw was green fields from the roof," she said.

Almost Missing the Bus in Italy

During fall break in October I went on an organized bus tour to Italy with my friend group. In Florence, I needed to meet the tour group in a city square after an afternoon of exploring on my own.

Not wanting to rush to find the meeting spot, I planned ahead and got to the square in advance of the scheduled meeting time and took the time to rest. As the time to meet the group grew closer and I saw no one I knew, I worried, *I'm in the wrong square!* This was prior to the widespread use of cell phones or GPS devices. *I have to figure out how to get back fast. They'll leave without me and return to the hotel. I don't know how to get there, it's outside the city. I'll be stranded in Florence.*

Using a paper map and asking people in my rudimentary Italian, "*Dove la chiesa* [where is the church]?" I found my way to the correct square, but I had to run. This was tricky because I couldn't run far or fast. When I finally arrived at the square, I saw everyone. *Thank goodness they waited for me and they don't even know about my heart.*

"Where have you been?" Karen asked. "Are you okay? Is something wrong? We've been so worried!"

"We begged the tour director to wait for you," Jeff said.

On the walk back to the bus, I breathlessly said to the tour director, "I'm so, so sorry! I have a heart condition and I couldn't run any faster."

"It's all right," he said to me. To the group on the bus he said, "Emily has a heart condition, so I waited, but I won't be doing that for anyone else again because her tardiness has had a great impact on our itinerary!"

Holding back tears as I sat, still trying to catch my breath, I thought, *I'm glad my heart got me out of this. I'm so embarrassed. My crappy navigation skills were the problem, not my heart.* I felt my cheeks turning red. *I'm going to have to factor in my heart to get places on time, or this is going to keep happening.* I replayed the tour director's speech in my head. *I can't face looking at anyone. How could he reveal my medical problems without even asking me?* I sneaked a look at my friend across the aisle. *I hope things don't change between us, now that she knows.* My friends on the bus didn't question me and I was glad not to have to explain. *What if this is not the only time I'll have to tell people about my heart to get out of something?*

Family Visit

When my family came to visit for Thanksgiving, Sam and I attended my first concert. We went to Wembley Stadium for an S Club 7 show. "It's so loud!" I said. All the children were blowing whistles.

"They don't do this at concerts at home," Sam said. I tried to block out the noise to hear the singing voices.

The following day, we went shopping together in my favorite greeting-card store near school. I grabbed Sam's arm and pulled her to the corner of the store. "Look!" I pointed. "It's Helena Bonham Carter, one of my favorite actresses." *I can't believe it's her! We both like the same store.*

"Cool," Sam said.

"We'll wait for her to finish shopping and then we're pouncing!" I said.

As Helena opened the door to leave the store, Sam and I approached her. "Hi, I'm Emily. You're in my favorite movie, and we watched your performance and analyzed it in my Shakespeare class today." She smiled and posed for a picture with both of us in front of her car, telling me she knew my teacher.

Spring Semester

Second semester, my friend group had returned to New Hampshire, so I spent most of my free time after school alone. I walked throughout London, for long distances but not at a fast pace, to see all the sights. It was fun to hear all the accents around me, smell the fish and chips baking in the pubs I passed, and become familiar with the different neighborhoods. *I don't need a map. I know what I'm doing now, and I see how everything connects,* I thought as I looked into the River Thames. *I'm getting the hang of this.*

Instead of traveling with friends on the weekends, I went to visit my European friends on my own. A British friend from home who studied in Massachusetts for her sophomore year of high school was living in Strasbourg, France. She lived in a picturesque house on the river, which was featured on many postcards. It was a white house with brown timber cutouts on the outside that made it look like a fairytale home.

"I'm so glad you're here," Charlie said. "I haven't seen you since we were eighteen and you visited me in Munich."

"That was the best trip, and the first and only time I've been drunk! That beach party together was so much fun, even though I puked that night," I said.

She laughed. "Don't drink too much French wine."

"No way, I learned my lesson." *I don't want to ever feel that way again.*

"I made quiche, let's eat. We can go touring tomorrow," she said.

It was January, cold and snowy, but we had a great time walking around the city, seeing the giant cathedral. We also saw the home to the European Parliament in a large circular building that reflected onto the water next to it.

Auntie came to visit me in London, and we spent the weekend in Barcelona. It was February and freezing cold, so we took a bus tour around town rather than walking. We saw some buildings that had been used in the Olympics and the architect Antoni Gaudí's work. We visited the church of the Sagrada Família, a mismatched, unfinished masterpiece. *Ugh, so many stairs. At least it's cold and not hot out.* I walked around the church, always finding new things to look at, tired after all the stairs. The passageways were narrow, and it was hard to find a place to rest, but Auntie and I found a corner on the roof where we saw the Barcelona skyline.

"It's so nice, and goes on forever," she said.

I was amused to see that not only did they sell fashion magazines on the main streets in the city, but they also sold live birds in cages. The tiny yellow birds squawked loudly for every passerby as they fluttered around in their brass cages, with little feathers littering the sidewalks. I stood watching them. *They smell, but it's cool they're for sale like this. It's so easy to get a pet bird here.* Dinner was always late in Spain, past nine or ten, and some of the dishes featured shrimp with their eyes still intact. "I can't eat this. It's looking at me!" I shoved the plate to Auntie. *The beady eyes are staring at me.* "I'll have melon and ham."

My Belgian friend from fall semester, who lived a few rooms away from me in the dorm, invited me to her home. One weekend in February, we traveled together to Brussels to see her family and explore her city. In the town square, she pointed out a bronze fountain sculpture of a tiny boy. "It's Manneken Pis. He's famous and he wears different hats and outfits depending on the season." I laughed and took his picture. We continued walking and I tried a chocolate-covered waffle. Later, we dined at a fancy restaurant where I indulged in a plate of vegetables that were luxuriously drowning in butter. *I feel like a princess eating this.*

Spring break, I visited with my family friends the Gees in France for a week. They live outside of Paris in a medium-sized city and are always welcoming and exciting to be with. We visited many castles together with green gardens full of sweet-smelling flowers and luxurious castle interiors. The Gees served delicious home-cooked meals, and I watched French fashion shows on TV. I also took the high-speed train into Paris for a day trip and walked around many neighborhoods endlessly, eating chocolate-filled croissants until I took the return train back.

"Let's go for a walk in the park," Phillipe said on our last day together. "First we'll stop at the market and get some turnips."

Hmm, I wonder why we're doing that. We always have fun, so I'll go along with this. We got the turnips and went to a farmhouse in the park.

Phillipe whistled quietly and a gray donkey lumbered out of the barn.

"Ah! I can't believe it! *Quelle surprise* [What a surprise]!" I said, running up to the gate to pet it.

"Give it some turnips, it will let you feed it," he said. Its hairy lips tickled my palms as I tried to think of French words the donkey might understand.

In April, my parents and Sam came to visit me, and we went to Scotland. After a full day of touring, we went shopping on the main street. In a Scottish-themed store, Sam and I tried on kilts and tam-o'-shanters. We posed for Mom, who took our picture as we pretended to dance around the dressing room.

Returning Home

In May, as my plane took off, I watched England get smaller and smaller and disappear beneath the clouds. I grinned, feeling healthy and strong after all of my walking around the city.

My seatmate, an Englishman, grinned back and asked, "Is this your first time to Boston?"

"No, I'm from there." *I must've really changed, he thinks I'm British!* "But this last year I lived in London."

"And how did you find it? Are you glad to be going home?"

I opened my mouth and closed it again, not sure where to start. "I had adventures ..."

Last Semester of School

In September, I went back to my mundane life at school in New Hampshire for my final semester before graduation in December 2003. I didn't have many friends, and I missed my London friend group. I returned to my old habit of mostly staying in my dorm room watching television and messaging with Mabel, who was away at college in Washington, DC.

I had a three-day school week and needed to build up my resume before graduation. I decided to keep my summer job at a department store in Boston on my long weekends. I traveled back and forth between school and home every week.

Mabel texted, "I'm going to a party at the frat house this weekend. Are you doing anything like that?"

"No, I've got work," I wrote.

"That's too bad. They're fun and you meet lots of guys!" she said.

"Maybe I can come visit you after graduation and go with you."

"Yeah, you shouldn't miss it."

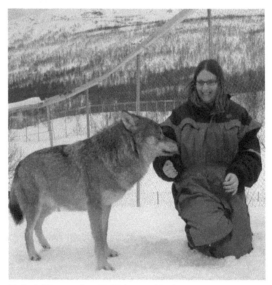

Emily in Norway, Age 29 (February 2012)

Everything Happens for a Reason

After college graduation, I moved back to Boston and lived at my parents' home for a while working at temporary jobs. Sam was in high school and we spent a lot of time together. Although she never exercised or played sports unless they were required in gym class, during her senior year of high school she joined the track team. I always had a sneaking suspicion that she felt guilty about being physically active, so I encouraged her not to hold back on my account. Whenever I saw her and her friends wearing their blue uniforms, I felt envious of her chance to be competitive. I yearned for those same experiences, even though I had no idea what it felt like to be on a team. Sam gave me lengthy summaries of the meets I missed because of work commitments, but I went to as many as I could to be supportive. It wasn't exactly the same, but living vicariously through her, I felt some of the team spirit.

Cardiac Patient Group

In my early twenties, I had an appointment with Dr. Anderson, the new doctor working with Dr. Smith. I walked into Dr. Smith's familiar waiting room and sat in one of the hard black chairs. I was called into the EKG room, which was now Dr. Anderson's office.

"I know it's so small in here," she laughed. "But if you think this is small, wait till you have your EKG in the copy room."

I smiled. "Oh well, nothing we can do."

"So, what did you do this weekend?" she asked as she took my blood pressure and I noted her minimal jewelry and black, sleek shoulder-length hair.

"I watched TV, so not much, I guess," I said. "What about you?" *We're about the same age.*

"I took care of my daughter while my husband worked. Let's go see Dr. Smith now."

Dr. Anderson was full of promises and plans. A few years later, she asked me, "How would you feel about meeting once a month with other patients like you to talk about cardiac issues or have fun together outside of the hospital?"

I wonder if this'll be like Open Hearts Camp? "All right, I'll go." *I haven't met anyone else with a heart condition since I was thirteen, so it's worth a try.*

I met with the group a few times for meals, once in the hospital cafeteria and then downtown at restaurants in Boston.

"I once lived in Africa when I was married," a woman a couple of years older than me said.

How could she live somewhere else and leave her doctors? And how old was she when she got married? She's my age.

"I am now being considered for a heart and lung transplant."

I hope that doesn't happen to me.

"I had my first surgery as a teenager, and I'll have to have more in the future," said a blonde woman who was younger than me and worked as a chef in one of my favorite restaurants.

Wow. I wonder how she's strong enough to work all day on her feet and deal with such a stressful place? I'm glad I won't have to have surgery again. My memories wouldn't fade as an adult and I'd remember everything.

One of the group members asked, "I have no family in the area. Can someone take me to my echo next month and my doctor appointment to hear the results?"

That's too bad they can't rely on their family like I can.

Another woman said, "I'm no longer able to work and am on disability. I try to do art projects at home and sell them online when I'm up to it."

She's only a few years older than me. How terrible she can't work for the rest of her life. She'll never get her quality of life back.

Once in a while Dr. Anderson joined us at our meetings, but I found, as time went on, I did not enjoy our group's time together. When new members joined us, the lone male member in our group said, "Let's all go around the table and discuss our histories." The unspoken rule of this share was to try and impress the members with what each person had gone through with the biggest story with the most problems.

It's so annoying that all the chronically ill people always compete, wherever we are. This group is fun when we don't talk about medical things, but I don't want to do this anymore. I left after only half a year.

Pilonidal Cysts

In 2006, at the age of twenty-four, I landed a full-time job in the travel industry and moved into my own apartment for the first time. The stress of living on my own and working full time took a toll on me. My body showed signs of stress and I developed pilonidal cysts. These cysts occur above the tailbone and are extremely painful, making it difficult to sit. They are unpredictable and can occur several times in a short period or remain dormant for months without incident. There is no way to prevent cysts from forming, except by undergoing preventive surgery that involves removing the area where cysts tend to grow. When I had an occurrence, the pain was so severe that it caused my body to shake, and I stayed home from work.

Pilonidal cysts continually grow and, unfortunately, the pus has to come to the surface before they can be treated. This might take several days. Once they are ready, a surgeon will lance them in the office. Because I experienced many recurrences, I required treatment frequently and went through three surgeons at three different hospitals in one year. This experience taught me how to advocate for myself. The first surgeon who treated my cyst at MGH fit all the doctor stereotypes I detested. He was cold, showy, and impersonal, which intimidated me, and I did not respond well to his personality. After he treated my cyst, he left me bleeding, face down on the exam table in a room by myself. I instantly decided I would never see this man again.

To switch doctors, I also switched hospitals. I went to the hospital where I was born, seeking the preventive surgery to stop future cysts from forming. The rigid doctor said, "I'm not performing this procedure on you. General anesthesia can be a concern for cardiac patients because it slows the heart rate. There are too many risks because of your cardiac history."

"Yes, I'm aware, but I need this surgery." I left the office thinking, *I'll change hospitals and surgeons, again.*

"Hi, I'm Doctor Toby." The new surgeon shook my hand. "Tell me what's going on?"

I explained my history. "Would you be willing to perform the surgery? I know it's risky and I haven't had anesthesia since I was six."

"Yes, I don't think it's a problem. We need to stop these cysts. If they continue to recur we will schedule the procedure," he said.

After several occurrences, ahead of my turning twenty-five in 2007, he operated and removed the area causing these cysts. Afterward, I came home and lay on my stomach on the hard floor, in a drugged haze, petting Benny. I stayed out of work for three days, and my recovery went well.

At home during my cyst surgery recovery, I was reading and I noticed that the letters on the page of my book were suddenly blurry.

I went to my postop checkup. "Dr. Toby, I've never had an eye problem before. What's going on?"

"That's odd," he said. "Maybe your pain killers are causing it. I'll call the ophthalmology department. Go there for an exam and further tests."

All the tests came back normal. For many years I noticed my eyes seemed a bit off, but I didn't have any more eye exams scheduled after the initial tests. I didn't realize more was needed to care for my eyes; nevertheless, I remained concerned about my vision.

Advocate for Yourself

"Dr. Smith, can I please see a different cardiologist?" I whispered. *Don't yell at me. Don't say I can't come here any longer. I'm not trying to be a burden.*

"You don't want to see Dr. Anderson anymore?"

"No. I know I can't be cured and we need to manage my problems forever, so I'd like to see another doctor who might be a better fit." *Changing doctors worked for my cyst.*

Dr. Cole, the newest cardiologist in Dr. Smith's practice, became my doctor in my late twenties and still is today. Whereas Dr. Smith was more authoritative and cautious, Dr. Cole and I have developed a rapport that works for us with two-way open and honest communication. At one of our first appointments together, she brought up something about my condition and I stopped her. "I don't know what you're talking about. I've been in the dark for twenty years." I stared at her hair tied back in a bun and her fancy jewelry. *You can do this. She's close to my age. There's nothing to be afraid of. She's nice. Get some answers. She's always excited about things. You can talk to her.*

"In the dark?" she asked.

I sighed, embarrassed. "I understand my condition only in child-like terms. Dr. Smith never really explained it to me in a way

I could understand. Doctors always said my condition was too rare to have a name. It was only when I started driving and started wearing a MedicAlert necklace that Sam looked up the words on the internet and we found the name of my condition."

Dr. Cole smiled and explained the parts of the heart to me and how mine functioned differently than other people's. "ALCAPA is a very rare condition. It stands for anomalous origin of the left coronary artery from the pulmonary artery. Here's what's important to understand: your left coronary artery came from the pulmonary artery instead of the aorta. Why is that important? The blood in the pulmonary artery goes to the lungs for oxygen. It's oxygen-poor blood. The blood in your aorta is oxygen-rich blood. The blood in your left coronary artery feeds your heart tissue. If there's not enough oxygen, tissue can die. Your heart compensated for the lack of oxygen by creating collateral arteries to feed oxygenated blood to your heart tissue and this enabled you to live as long as you did. But it wasn't enough oxygen and you suffered a heart attack. You also have mitral valve regurgitation. This is why you had to have surgery as a young child. Your mitral valve still leaks even though you have the ring, because that doesn't prevent it completely. Do you sort of understand a little now?"

I shrugged. *That's a lot.*

"Do you have more questions?" Dr. Cole asked.

I thought for a moment, having never been asked this before, and I said hesitantly, "Do you know anything about my life expectancy or if I can ever have a baby?"

"I can't answer about life expectancy, since many people haven't survived this long with your history. The medicine you're on will keep your heart working less now so it will be stronger later. As for having babies, it's possible you could carry one. When the time comes, we can discuss it more."

As time went on, I saw Dr. Cole more and Dr. Smith less and less. He was still an email away. Although I was sad, I was reassured in case anything unexpected came up.

Preparing for Japan

When I was twenty-eight, in 2010, an annual physical revealed issues with my eyesight, just a week before a long-awaited trip to Japan. On my trips around the world, I genuinely thrive. I try never to stay home when I can go somewhere new, living by my motto of "Don't waste a second." I plan epic vacations for myself and usually travel alone, unafraid to travel independently, without a companion. I am less reserved and open to more experiences, such as flying in a small plane to land on a glacier, participating in animal encounters, or finding my way to a remote place to see something unusual. Vacation frees me from appointments and proximity to dreaded medical places. It can also be the light at the end of the tunnel when I'm going through an arduous medical situation and need something positive to hold onto. Trips also give me confidence in myself, knowing I can handle my medical struggles away from Boston and get by on my own. I research contact information for physicians at each destination and then my doctors give me permission to go.

The day of my physical the doctor sent me to an eye specialist to further investigate my problems. *Is Japan still happening?*

At the ophthalmology appointment, the technician did an eye pressure test and right away found the pressure was extremely high.

"You have glaucoma," the technician said. "Glaucoma is a condition of increased pressure within the eye. It causes a gradual loss of sight. There's no cure for this condition. You can only try to manage it."

"Okay. Can I still go to Japan?" I asked.

"Yes," the ophthalmologist said. "But you should go to Massachusetts Eye and Ear Infirmary when you return from Japan for specialist care. You can go back to work today."

What a relief. I'm so happy I can still go.

I arrived back at my office at 2 p.m., and at 2:10 p.m., the Mass Eye and Ear glaucoma department called, shrieking at me, "It's essential that you come in right away!"

Nervous, I quickly gathered my belongings at work and took the twenty-minute subway ride to the new hospital. I had eye tests from 2:30 to 5:30 p.m. that Friday. When I met Dr. Knight, my newly assigned glaucoma specialist, I had no idea what to expect after an afternoon of testing. Dr. Knight did another eye-pressure test and the results were shocking to her. "A normal eye pressure range is around ten to twenty-one and your eye is at sixty-six! I've never seen any pressure that high. You've permanently lost some vision in your right eye because it's damaged the optic nerve."

My mouth dropped open in shock. *How could I not know? When my eyes are open, I don't see anything differently.* I closed my left eye to check the vision in the right. *Oh, I guess I do see honeycombs where my vision should be clear.*

"Because your blind spot overlaps with the left eye, you didn't realize how serious this has become. Also, I think it's why this hasn't been discovered until now," Dr. Knight said.

She let me know I had chronic angle-closure glaucoma. I got to know her soft-spoken, kind demeanor. She told me, "Immediate action is necessary to prevent further vision loss. We have to get your eye pressure down to the twenties by Monday. If it doesn't get lower, we will start you on medication and there probably will be no trip to Japan at the end of the week. Instead, I think you'll need surgery to help lower the pressure. Your vision might decrease, but without me performing the surgery, you could go blind."

This was a lot to take in. But, unlike other surgeons, she spoke quietly, as if she didn't feel she had to yell to demonstrate her superiority, which made me more confident in trusting her to perform the surgery.

ICE

The beginning of the week after my diagnosis, I saw a cornea specialist. He asked, "Do you have herpes? Many types of glaucoma are caused by that virus. If you have it or get it, it could affect both of your eyes."

"No." I said, completely embarrassed at the thought. *Great, now I have another thing to be terrified of for life.*

After a negative herpes test and further testing, he diagnosed me with a variant of chronic angle-closure glaucoma, iridocorneal endothelial syndrome (ICE), a unique ophthalmic disorder that is one form of glaucoma. The doctor informed me about detrimental activities that could lead to bacteria entering my eye and damaging my vision, things as simple as the common cold.

So Long, Japan

Everything was happening so fast after my diagnosis that I didn't have time to research or worry about all the complications of potential eye surgery. I had other things to focus on.

I called Mabel. "I'm so angry. I don't want to lose more eyesight. I should've stood up for myself like you would, to push to get more diagnostic tests."

"But you couldn't pin down what was wrong," she said patiently.

"It's been four years, but I didn't know how bad the damage was or that it's permanent. Now I probably can't go to Japan and all my planning is down the drain."

"Don't worry, you can go when you get better. I wish we didn't have to deal with any of this and we could be carefree campers again," she said.

"Me too." I sighed.

For my first time as an adult, I experienced an urgent medical situation by myself, making everything more stressful. My parents and Sam were overseas on vacation at the time. I emailed my parents to update them on what was going on. Mom wrote back, "Sorry that yet more crap is piled on you ..." Sam managed to find a pay phone and called me early one morning, afternoon for her, and we chatted for a while. During the call, I felt less alone.

The week of my departure, I returned to see Dr. Knight for the second time and she confirmed, "Instead of flying to Japan on Friday, you'll be having eye surgery the following Monday." I went home to modify my already packed suitcase for a recovery stay at my parents' home after surgery. I felt oddly calm. *I don't know what to expect, so there's nothing to be afraid of. I have to save my eyesight.*

Eye Surgery Recovery

In late October 2010, Dr. Knight performed my first eye surgery. Mom, Dad, and Sam sat in the waiting room while I was awake and under local anesthesia. Dr. Knight created a new drainage site in my eye to lower the eye pressure. After a few hours, I went back to my childhood home wearing an eye shield to recover. I knew I couldn't stay home alone since I didn't know how much pain I'd be in or how capable I'd be of taking care of myself.

Bright light caused me pain. I kept my head under blankets and kept the shades drawn to shield my eyes. *I'm like a vampire, so sensitive to light.* I listened to TV shows with my eyes closed and didn't read. When some light streaked in, or I'd hear loud noises that made me blink in reflex, I'd shout, "Turn those off! It hurts!" The pain was short-lived, but sharp enough to make me yell.

Living at home with my parents took some getting used to. *I miss the city. I feel like a kid again.*

"Emily, did you do your lunch-time drops?" Mom asked as I sat down at the table to eat a sandwich.

"Yes," I sighed. *She's monitoring me so closely.*

Every morning Dad and I went for a short walk around the neighborhood; every evening Mom made dinner and we ate together as a family. *It's nice to all be together, but I miss eating my chocolates and waking up late at my house. I guess it's nice not making choices and having everyone take care of me. I shouldn't complain.*

My family also helped me with the activities I was restricted from, such as lifting heavy items, bending over, and driving. I had to squat rather than bend, which meant spitting out toothpaste in the sink with my head held upright and picking things up from the floor with a grabber stick. In the shower, I wore glasses that had a sponge on the top rim to try to keep water out of my eyes. My parents drove me to my postop checkups and any other appointments I had scheduled.

Every day I administered stinging eye drops. I stood in the bathroom and tilted my head up and squeezed the liquid in. It burned and my eye gushed tears, but I didn't cry. My family would hear me if I cried or shouted and I didn't want to distress anyone. I quietly stamped my foot and wiped my tears away with a tissue.

One morning, when I came out of the bathroom, I passed Sam in the hall and she said, "Your eye's red. Does it hurt?"

"No, it's always red," I replied nonchalantly and walked into the kitchen where Dad was eating breakfast.

"How are you feeling today?" he asked.

"Fine. Same as before." I joined him at the table, blinking to conceal the pain.

"I'll come with you to your checkup at Dr. Knight's this week." Dad had been at work during the majority of my checkups and procedures after my first open-heart surgery. It took some getting used to, having him accompany me to my medical appointments now that he was retired, but it was a welcome change.

"Great," I happily replied and started to think of things to do together near the appointment so we could get more out of our downtown Boston outing.

When Dad finished breakfast, he went for a walk and Mom returned from her daily four-mile walk and came to my room to check on me.

"How are you doing?"

My stoic act didn't work on Mom. "My drops hurt a lot and my head hurts from the eye pain."

She nodded. As she had experienced her own medical problems for most of her life, I never worried she'd overreact to my discomfort.

It can take from one to three months to fully heal after eye surgery, but most activities can be resumed much sooner. I returned to my condo after two weeks and work after three weeks. I wore sunglasses whenever I left the house to protect my eyes from incoming debris. This was a temporary solution until my eye healed. I had not worn eyeglasses or contacts previously, but eventually I would start wearing prescription glasses to aid my vision, which had decreased from the surgery, and to protect my good eye.

At work, I sat at the reception desk and walk-in visitors made several hurtful jokes and comments about the sunglasses I was wearing. "Is it too bright in here for you? Are you working at the beach? Are you a movie star trying to conceal your appearance? What are you hiding?" *I can't react, or I'll get fired.* I cried about the comments later, when I returned home.

Confiding in a Friend

"I had the worst day," I texted Mabel.

"What happened?"

"I went glasses shopping for the first time. The glasses in the store were screaming at me like bandages or a cast on a hurt limb. They're announcing a visual sign of disability to the world. I can't hide my problem."

"I've always had glasses. No one thinks that. Get over it, it's not a big deal," she said.

"You're much tougher than me. I don't think like that. I thought I'd get them when I'm older and I'm not ready to have them yet."

"You won't think like that after a few months, I bet."

"I hope so," I said. "At least I can take them off when I get home every day."

"Did you go to that party with your work friends?"

"No. I don't want to drive at night anymore. The headlights from oncoming traffic blind me. And there's no bus to where they live."

"Oh, no. That stinks."

"I had this headlight problem before the surgery and I thought it'd go away, but it's still happening so no more night driving for now."

"It's too bad about the party, but you'll get another chance," she said.

"They're such a fun group and we were just starting to be better friends. And while I'm complaining, I also can't bend much or tilt my head down. It puts too much pressure on my eye, so I can't pick stuff up without squatting."

"There's so much you have to remember to do now," she said.

I sighed, even though she couldn't hear me over text.

Japan and Singapore

"The wait is finally over." Dr. Knight said. "You've been patient for six months since the surgery, and now it's safe for you to travel."

"Great! Dr. Cole said I could go, too. I'll go to Japan and Hong Kong," I said. *I can't wait to be free from all these appointments and get away from the hospital. I'm still going to be adventurous and able to travel with my heart and eye. I'm not going to have to give up traveling!*

In April 2011, I checked the morning news online and I gasped. *An earthquake and tsunami in Japan!* I saw a news report in Japan with a reporter who filmed the action in real time. As the journalist stumbled, the video image flipped as if the world was turning and everything was upside down. *That's terrible! Especially for all of my friends there!* I emailed my friends to check on them. *I'm supposed to leave in two weeks. There's no way I can go to Japan now.* Disappointed, I scanned flights for a new city near Hong Kong to change my plane ticket to. *I remember Jack went to Singapore and he said they have a great zoo. I'll check it out.*

I changed my ticket to Hong Kong and Singapore and departed a few weeks later. In Hong Kong, I met up with my friend June, whom I had met when she lived in Boston for a year.

"Emily, I want you to meet baby Ava." She handed me her four-month-old baby to hold.

"She's so cute. She's got so much hair!" I said as I bounced her on my knee.

"I'm glad you got to meet her. If you'd come in October, I would've still been pregnant."

"It all worked out," I said.

In Hong Kong, I went to see the Big Buddha, Tian Tan, in Lantau. *Oh my gosh, I have to climb 268 stairs to reach him.* Walking extremely slowly and taking numerous rest breaks, I didn't give up. *I'm going to make it, no matter how long it takes. I have all day, no one's waiting for me.* I enjoyed looking around at the scenery on my twenty-minute journey up. I saw bright blue skies shining above me as I trudged up the stairs, with beautiful flowers along the way. There were many shades of blue in the clear sky and I was relieved I could still see them and everything else around me. The tourists, including me, took many selfies with the Buddha and I met people who took my photo for me despite the language barrier.

When I went to the Orangutan Breakfast at the Singapore Zoo, there were large red-orange-colored orangutans, including a small baby, sitting on a platform. Visitors, including me, could stand in front of the platform and take pictures with them. We could not touch them owing to the risk of spreading disease but could stand at a close angle for photos. The orangutans stayed on the platform by choice because they had plenty of juicy green leaves to eat. I stood with my back to them for the picture and I could feel them moving their sticks and large leaves around as they brushed my arms, back, and head. I heard them chewing and rustling the leaves as they waved their branches near my face and eyes while I posed for the photos. *Don't touch my eyes, I don't want to go to the doctor.* I smiled and stood still for the photos, because it was a risk I wanted to take.

During my week in Singapore, I explored as much as time allowed. Visiting the four distinct areas of town—Chinese, Malay, Indian, and Eurasian—I had a great time. I loved seeing the colorful fabrics, hearing the languages, and eating the exotic foods. It was like traveling to India, China, and the Middle East without ever leaving Singapore. Despite locals cautioning me not to eat the spicy food, I persisted and surprised them by loving it. Even with my mouth burning, I always went back for more.

In the mornings after eating too much at the breakfast buffet, I went to the pool at my hotel. While lying on my white lounge chair in the humid air, I often heard the street sweepers on the road below, as they were constantly making Singapore shine. It was a very clean city and evidence of the care taken was everywhere, with no litter to be seen. I also heard tropical birds in the trees, since I was high up on the rooftop, but sweepers beeping away was the most common sound. I didn't go into the water above my shoulders, cautious about getting water in my eye, but I was glad to take that first step into reclaiming something fun.

Trying new things never tired me out, but the heat was draining. It was humid, moist, and uncomfortable outside every day, all day. The humidity was easily forty to fifty percent higher than it would have been in Boston. On the sixth day of my trip, I hit my limit and sought refuge in air conditioning. I opted to spend the day at a mall, enjoying an Indian film with English subtitles in a reserved theater seat, which was a novel experience for me. The movie, a musical love story about a robot's companionship with a college-aged woman, featured singing and dancing numbers and colorful costumes in bright reds, golds, and yellows. The dancers wore shiny bangles on their wrists. Although I didn't understand the language, I downloaded the upbeat songs upon returning home and happily sang along.

Walking to the subway station from my hotel, and seeing the National Heart Center and the Singapore National Eye Center directional signs, made me smirk each day. *It's ironic that both my problems are treated in the same place. Probably a good thing if I need to know where to go. Do other people commonly have both problems together?* I looked at the driveway but never saw any patients or staff going in or out of the big white buildings. *It's so hot. I'm walking like a snail ... Oh phew, there's the station. Can't wait for the air conditioning.* After two weeks away with no significant health issues, the eye surgery was behind me. *I'm ready to face whatever's next.*

The Second Eye Surgery

At my appointment with Dr. Knight after my return from Asia she said, "The body likes to heal things. You've grown new tissue over the surgical drain which has covered the hole. Your pressure's gone up again."

For the next six months, I was in a state of limbo with many appointments.

"This week we'll try these drop combinations. Your pressure's still too high to come off of the other one," Dr. Knight said.

Another trip to the pharmacy tonight.

"Your pressure's still too high," Dr. Knight said. "We've been trying for several months now to control it with medication but it's not working. We're going to have to do another surgery. I'm going to need to implant a permanent shunt tube to drain your eye to lower the pressure."

"Will it be visible?" I asked.

"No, I'll put it under your eyelid," Dr. Knight replied.

Phew. I don't care then. "Okay, we can do it." *I'm glad we have a plan now so I don't have to wonder what's going to happen at every appointment anymore.*

The surgery in September 2011 was similar to the first one almost a year prior. My parents came with me for support, but Sam was away at school. The main difference with this surgery was the IV. Unlike the previous one, when they had placed it relatively easily, this time, despite several attempts to insert the IV into my arm veins, the doctors couldn't place the line at all. When the anesthesiologist arrived and stood next to me while I lay on the gurney, I pointed to my arm and said, "This vein works best. The others are much worse, so that's your best shot."

The anesthesiologist thought he knew better than me, however, and refused to listen. He didn't attempt to use my good vein and proceeded to poke and prod me on both arms with no success.

"Let's try to use your hand," he said.

I haven't done that since I was six. I tried to stop this from happening, crying, "Please don't do it, try anywhere else. I can take it."

The doctor gave in and said, "Okay, we'll try your foot."

Damn, but better than my hand.

"You have to go down to the children's surgical floor because those anesthesiologists are more practiced with foot insertion."

Dr. Knight came into the children's room to supervise since preparations were taking much longer than usual.

"Don't worry, Emily. We'll get the IV in. It'll work," she said as she held my hand.

I closed my eyes as the cold rubbing alcohol they applied to my foot evaporated. After two tries, the needle went in successfully with minimal pain. *I can't see anything so I can pretend it's not my foot. There's no IV here.*

In the children's holding room where I waited to go into the operating room, a young child was preparing for his surgery as well.

I looked over at the little boy in the same blue and white hospital gown as me, sitting up on his gurney under a white blanket, holding his mom's hand, and we smiled at each other. A short while later, I was wheeled into the operating room.

As with the previous surgery, doctors gave me a nerve block to ensure that I wouldn't feel anything, but I still had to remain awake and aware throughout the surgery. While Dr. Knight worked, I mouthed the words to a Lady Gaga song playing on the radio. My eye was covered with a cloth, but I could see flashes of light sometimes, although nothing in detail. Every so often I could start to feel things and had to say, "I feel something pulling." Dr. Knight administered local numbing medications and I'd go back to listening to the radio.

A few hours after the procedure ended, I was ready to return home. I went to my parents' house where they took care of me. *Light doesn't hurt this time and I remember the care routine. But my pain's worse. I guess it's the stitches securing the implant.* The stitches irritated the insides of my eyelid and felt like sand granules on fire. *At least it's not constant, but it hurts depending on where my eyeball moves.* I tried to sleep during the worst of it and took pain killers when needed. I could no longer rub my eye because of the delicate nature of the implant. *Ugh, my vision's worse. I'll have to get new glasses again and I'll have to wear them all day, constantly. I can't take them off at home anymore.*

The next morning, I stood at the bathroom sink and administered the first of five drops for the day. *I have to know what time it is, so I don't miss a scheduled dose. I can't go anywhere without planning ahead in case I'm without the drops.* I mentally checked off my first drop on the daily schedule, propped up on the bathroom sink.

During my postop checkups, Dr. Knight found she was not getting the results she wanted for my eye pressure. "Your implant is not working as effectively as I hoped. Your pressure's still high."

She paused. "It's not uncommon in ICE syndrome to need more than one tube implant."

I guess I can get through it, we need to save my eye.

"You can't return full-time to work in three weeks. You can only return part-time," Dr. Knight said. I resumed living on my own and every day after work I returned home to rest my eye.

Postsurgical Eye Checkups

I went to see Dr. Knight every other week, to check my eye pressure and decide when she could clear me to return to work full-time. *Wow! They really love soap operas. This is the fourth episode in a row they've shown.* Time went by slowly during the one-to-four-hour wait.

I'll close my eyes. I'm so tired ...

"It's my turn! How much longer do I have to wait?" an older woman patient shouted at the passing technician.

My eyes popped open.

"A while," Nolan, the technician replied. "There's many people ahead of you."

"This is ridiculous. We shouldn't have to wait so long!" she snapped to her husband.

I rolled my eyes. *Dr. Knight's the best, so I won't complain. I'm good at waiting for doctors.*

While most of my eye checkups consisted of long boring waits, in October something fun happened.

"Hi, Emily," Kerri, one of the technicians, said while I waited. "How are you? Let me see your nails this week!"

Smiling, I showed Kerri my hand. "Some green sparkles."

"Come with me!" she said, and I followed her into the staff locker room.

"Sit here on the bench and I'll draw a ghost on your nail," Kerri said. She pulled out her nail paints.

"Thank you so much ... ooh, I love the black eyes. It's perfect for Halloween."

Afterward, I went back to the waiting room. Bored and nervous, I returned to reading the book I brought along, but I couldn't concentrate. *I have no idea how my eye's doing. I can't feel any change in pressure.*

"Emily, we can take you back now," called Nolan.

Following him to the back of the office, I entered a semi-dark room and sat down in the center chair. *I hate answering all of these history questions and remembering when I took my drops.*

"Please read the largest letters you see on the chart," he said.

"A, K, maybe L ...," I responded.

"Okay. Come with me into the next room and wait for Dr. Knight."

I followed Nolan to the new room and sat in the chair with a tall back and footrest.

Dr. Knight came into the room a short while later and kindly asked as she closed the door, "How's your eye feeling?"

"It's okay, but I've noticed a few things," I said.

"Let's check your pressure."

Scooching forward in my chair, I rested my chin on the chin rest on the slit lamp, an instrument Dr. Knight used to examine my eye. She sat across from me and lifted my upper eyelid, since I always have trouble keeping it open. My lashes hit the machine and I sat back, blinked, and came forward again to restart.

Dr. Knight tapped her ear and said, "Look at my earring."

I wonder what earring Dr. Knight will have this week? Maybe the usual tiny square diamond stud. I love this game, like I used to play with Mrs. Neth.

A blue light shone into my eye and she took a pressure reading while I stared straight ahead. She measured both eyes. Trying to stay still for the five seconds the test took was a challenge. *This is so uncomfortable. I want it to end!*

When I squirmed and kicked my foot, Dr. Knight asked, "Are you okay? You're doing a great job."

"Yes." I held my breath in anticipation of bad news.

After checking the pressure, Dr. Knight looked at the back of my eye to examine the optic nerve and check for any other issues. She made sure the tube was still in the correct place and working. Dr. Knight sat back at her desk away from the instruments and told me the results. "You've developed a cyst near your implant again. You know it's a common thing that can happen after surgery. The cyst has reformed and needs to be drained. We need to do eye needling, like we did two weeks ago."

"Sure, no problem." *Anything's better than doing this with an IV in the OR.* "I'd rather do this again," I said.

Dr. Knight gave me some numbing drops and I sat still in the chair looking at the floor. Dr. Knight lifted my eyelid and poked the cyst straight on to pierce it and drain it.

I feel nothing and it's drained. I can go home.

Gathering my things, I left the office. Outside, I called my family on a conference call and reported on the office gossip. "I had a Dr. Knight appointment. Nolan told me about his kids."

"How are they?" Dad asked.

"His son—"

"What's your eye pressure?" Sam interrupted.

She hates hearing about the staff. Now I'll have to tell everyone and disappoint them.

"Twenty. That's still too high for me because of the damage I already have so the goal is the high to mid-teens."

"What did Dr. Knight say to do?" Mom asked.

"Come back in two weeks," I said, discouraged.

Months later, in early February 2012, I had a different post-checkup report for my family. I stood outside freezing and called them. "I had a Dr. Knight appointment. All the drop combinations we've been trying finally worked!"

"Whoa!" Dad laughed. "That's great news!"

"It only took a year and a half since my diagnosis!" I said. "Dr. Knight said that the pressure might go up again and I might need another surgery, but for now I'm okay."

Magical Ice Holiday

Prior to glaucoma, I'd never faced opportunities being taken away because of anything other than my heart. After my second eye surgery, I decided not to let moments be denied before they have to be. *Another eye surgery's looming. I'm not going to keep waiting to live my life.* I went to the library to research new travel destinations. I've been lucky to have the resources to travel. I worked at my job long enough that I did not lose income from my time out of office because of illness. Trying not to spend money on things I don't need throughout the year, I save for trips and cut costs in other ways when possible. On vacations, I enjoy simple food and accommodations in order to budget for experiences instead.

In late February, my eye and heart were stable, so I booked a trip to Norway, which I called my "Magical Ice Holiday." This trip was significant to me as I had always wanted to visit there on my honeymoon and stay in a hotel made of ice or snow. *I'm not getting married anytime soon. Stop waiting for something that might never happen.* It was a record year for solar flares, so there was a good chance of seeing the northern lights. *I'd better go see them, before I might not be able to see them at all.*

Before boarding the plane from Oslo to Tromsø, the starting point for my Arctic adventure, I noticed a sign at another gate that read "Beware of polar danger." Svalbard, another destination, had more polar bears than people. *Add that to the to-do list for the future!* From the city center in Tromsø, I joined a tour that took me out to a deserted area with no city lights. Wearing my snow pants, along with several warm layers, I lay in the snow looking up at the green and yellow lights dancing in the sky. Sometimes small bursts of light shone in the darkness and other times light danced across the navy-blue sky reflecting in the lake below. Although some say you can hear the lights, I didn't. I heard only the silence around me.

While I was in the Arctic Circle, I went on reindeer and dog-sled rides, enjoying my time spent with animals. *I'm excited to go to the Polar Zoo tomorrow. I hope the language barrier doesn't cause problems on the bus.* When I couldn't communicate in English, I pointed to maps and printouts of where I wanted to go. The bus got me to the stop closest to the zoo and I hired a taxi for the remainder of the journey.

Playing with wolves and arctic foxes was the highlight of the trip. The giant tan-, white-, and black-haired wolves put their paws on my shoulders and tried to kiss me on the face many times. *No kisses allowed. No germs near my eye!* I turned my head to the side to avoid their generous kisses. One wolf peed on my leg to tag me as his own so the rest of the pack could not claim me. *I can't believe he likes me so much!* As I knelt during the encounter, two wolves fought right in front of me, rolling in the snow, baring their sharp white teeth and growling to display dominance. *My heart's racing. I forgot what it feels like when I'm excited.*

Last but not least, it was time for the main event. I went to the Snow Hotel at the top of the world, in Kirkenes. The hotel was like an igloo, a white dome-shaped structure with a dark arched opening and no windows. There were chairs lined up outside, similar to a beach for sun/snow gazing. Since the sun set early, the name "Snow Hotel" was projected in bright letters in the snow at the entrance so you could find your way back if you got lost walking around the property.

Inside, at a bar made of ice, a bartender offered warm drinks or a chance to sit on a chair made of ice under icicle chandeliers. A server announced, "Every year a different artist is selected to design the bedrooms. Inside each room different snow art is carved into the walls and there are ice sculptures."

I don't feel like sitting still. I'm going to look around the rooms before anyone claims the one I want. Wandering down the halls I looked into each room. I chose one with a swan ice sculpture and an image of an indigenous person etched into the wall behind the bed. The bed was a square block of ice with reindeer hides on top and a sleeping bag with snowflake-patterned flannel pillows.

After staking my claim I met the hospitality director across from the hotel in an unheated concrete building. "Luggage is not brought into the Snow Hotel. All activities like brushing your teeth, using the restroom, or changing clothes are done here. You can also return here during the night if you don't want to stay in your ice bed."

When it was time for bed, the hospitality director said, "Strip down to your leggings. They'll keep you warm. Wear this balaclava face mask."

I'll look like a bank robber, with only my eyes showing!

"Won't we get cold?" a guest asked.

"No. You don't need all of your clothing layers to stay warm since you'll all be in feather down sleeping bags."

I eagerly climbed into the bag and tucked myself in for the night, relishing the excitement of the experience. The insulated snow walls surrounding me created a deafening silence that drowned out any outside noise or neighbors. My breath filled the frigid air in front of me as I peeked out of the sleeping bag. The lights never shut off. During the night I woke up many times and tossed and turned. Sometimes my mask slipped down and parts of my face were cold, but never my body. To ensure my eye drops didn't freeze, I kept them in a pouch attached to a necklace resting on my chest to preserve their liquid state with my body heat. The next morning, I woke up early, feeling somewhat tired but proud that I had made it through the night. Not all the other guests had stayed for the entire night at the Snow Hotel. My wish for a "Magical Ice Holiday" had come true, and it was time to head back home.

"Please fasten your seatbelts and put your trays up. We're getting ready for takeoff," the flight attendant said.

Looking down on Norway, I sighed. *I'll have to go back to seeing Dr. Knight all the time. This vacation was over too fast. I don't want to have another eye surgery.*

Bad Things Happen in Threes

"Will you tell me now why you've been so quiet?" I asked Mom on the phone when I got home from Norway. "You barely emailed me."

"Sam's doctor found a lump and she has thyroid cancer."

Oh no!

"But she's never been sick before," I said. "How could this be? Why didn't you tell me?"

"We didn't want to worry you. She's going to come home from school in DC to have a checkup here with her doctor in a few weeks to make a treatment plan. There's nothing we can do until then."

I hate being the non-sick person and waiting. I wish it was me who was sick instead. I know I could handle it. Sam was strong and would get through it, but I worried about how she would grapple with being the patient. Before Sam returned to school, we went out for a family dinner. At the table, she let us know what her doctor told her at her appointment earlier in the day.

"I need surgery to have my thyroid removed. I also have to have radiation afterward. I can do it here at MGH after the semester's over in early May."

We all silently picked at our food, trying to make conversation about other topics.

At my eye checkups my eye pressure continued to creep upward. Dr. Knight scheduled a third surgery for April 2012. She would put in another valve implant in the corner of my eye near my nose. This surgery was quite different from the first two. This time, it was Dad and me at the hospital on Monday morning. Mom was in the hospital recovering from her own recent unscheduled major surgery and Sam would be returning from school to have her surgery in two weeks. Both would be inpatients, but I would return home the same day. I couldn't rely on Dad for help as much as I did after the first two eye surgeries because he would soon have Mom and Sam needing help as well. *How's Dad going to handle this? I have to care for them and still remember to take care of me. This is so hard with three of us needing surgery within weeks of each other. I can't handle this by myself, I need help. It's unbelievable that we're all sick at the same time.*

I began speaking with a therapist, Tina, to get me through this troublesome period.

"I don't think I feel as much sympathy for Mom and Sam as I should. I'm jealous I'm not the only sick one. I'm a monster for saying it, but I miss the spotlight."

"What else are you feeling?"

"My family keeps their fear and pain hidden from each other. It's so tense."

"I'll give you some techniques and exercises to handle the stress and anxiety. They should help," Tina said.

Focus on the big picture, not the small details. Everything will get better, this is just temporary. I made food for myself, unlike during previous recoveries, and took care of myself without as much help. I set up medical supplies in Mom's and Sam's rooms, being sure to attend to their limitations. I put a bench in the shower so they could sit, and kept a grabber stick in the kitchen so we could pick things up without having to bend. I made them each welcome home signs that I put on their doors.

Before work, I visited Sam at MGH the day after her surgery. Reading in a chair outside of her room, I waited for her to wake up and then went in. We talked until I had to leave, around 8:30.

I returned after my part-time workday was over and helped Sam with her discharge instructions, and we went home. When Mom returned from the hospital, I made her lunch and got her medicine. It felt good to be there for my family when they really needed someone. I focused less on my pain while helping Mom and Sam. They weren't used to being on the receiving end of care, and I wasn't used to being the caregiver. There was some tension while we all negotiated playing different roles than we were used to. Just like any typical family, we had some arguments and challenges, but we pulled through it and healed. They have since recovered and have not needed additional surgeries.

Life with an Eye Condition

"There's no cure," Dr. Knight said at an appointment. "Going forward, we're going to try to manage your rare form of glaucoma, depending on what symptoms show up."

Even though more has been taken away from me, I have to see the positives. Something good has come out of every health hurdle I've ever experienced.

I want to take off my glasses forever and return to the face I used to have, but that will never happen. *If I only think about all my restrictions, I'll never get out of bed. Keep going. I'm lucky with the conditions I've been dealt. Concentrating on what I do have and can do is better than focusing on all I have lost. Being sick is my normal; feeling well is unusual and uncomfortable at times.*

Speak Up

Occasionally, I have to tackle both my heart and eye conditions at the same time. I have to prioritize the body part that needs my attention and make sure doctors understand that the two conditions are equally important and have the doctors work together. To get my point across when my eye is downplayed and all the attention is focused on my heart, I often say, "You can replace a heart, but not an eye." That usually stuns doctors into silence.

Sometimes Dr. Knight gives me an explanation about something common to her, but I don't understand what she means and she doesn't always explain the medical terms.

"Your bleb's doing well," she said at an appointment.

What's that? Don't stay quiet! I yelled at myself. *Speak up! You aren't wasting her time. You need to understand.*

"Can you remind me what that is?" I asked hesitantly.

"The bubble in the eye tissue that I made over the drain during surgery."

I have to be my own advocate to receive the best care and manage my body's upkeep and mental health.

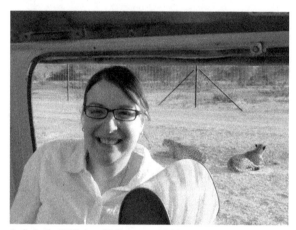

Emily in the UAE, Age 32 (February 2015)

Shocking Procedures

In May 2013, Sam and I went on a two-week vacation to Morocco, about a year after my last eye surgery and just before I turned thirty-one. We rode camels in the desert and visited souks (outdoor markets) with a colorful array of items for sale, including tin lanterns, leather goods, aromatic spices displayed in barrels, and silk blankets of all colors. I fell in love with Moroccan mint tea, a warm, extra-sweet drink full of sugar, served in glasses with intricate designs to welcome guests wherever we went. As we walked through narrow alleys, Sam and I heard the pounding of hooves and braying as dusty donkeys transported goods with their owners around the city. Sweat dripped down my neck almost all day, every day. We hurried to see as many major sites as possible, from Rabat to Marrakech. Even while resting in the car, we made sure not to miss anything. During one fun drive, we saw several goats in a tree, greedily eating argon nuts. Overall, we had a good trip, despite some hiccups, such as our luggage getting lost on the way home.

Sam and I arrived back in Boston on a Friday and that weekend, while staying with our parents, I became ill with a mild case of "traveler's tummy." I spent three days at my parents' house recuperating. While I was there, I worked on tracking down our luggage with the airlines. By Wednesday, our luggage was retrieved, and Sam had returned to her home in DC. I was back in my own home and feeling better, so I returned to work.

Suddenly, on Friday morning, one week after we returned, I woke up in the middle of the night with my heart beating extremely rapidly. It was pitch black and I was lying on my stomach. My first thought was of Miss Clavel from the *Madeline* book series, who famously said, "Something is not right!" Madeline was ill in the middle of the night, and her appendix ultimately needed to be removed, but I didn't know what was wrong with me. *I've never felt anything like this. My heart feels like it's dancing or that I've done something crazy active.*

I followed my first cardiologist's advice. Dr. Gold always told my parents, "Wait and see." He didn't believe in overreacting to situations that might change for the better if we gave them time. His words stay with me whenever I encounter something unexpected. I glanced at the clock: 4:13. Blood wasn't gushing out of me. I remained calm and went back to sleep.

I woke up to my alarm beeping three hours later and took the bus to my HR office. My heart was still beating irregularly but I didn't notice anything else on the walk to or from the bus stop or office. My manager knew about my heart condition, and I timidly went into her office prior to my other colleagues' arrival at nine. I said, "My heart's acting strangely and I don't know what to do. It's never happened before, but I don't feel bad other than that." *I don't want to be paranoid, but something's off. I know she won't be emotional about whatever this is and can tell me what to do objectively.*

After putting down her cell phone and turning to focus on me, she said, "I think you should go to the hospital. I can arrange a taxi and go with you."

"No, I want to take the subway." *I'd rather go alone.* "I'll get myself there, safely."

I stepped out of the office into the hallway. I called the cardiology office and the receptionist said, "Come in to see us."

On the twenty-minute subway ride, I stared at the Charles River hoping that Dr. Cole was in so that I didn't have to be examined by a stranger. When I arrived at the cardiology department, I went right to the reception desk. "Is Dr. Cole here?" I asked.

"No, she's not. But Dr. Smith is here consulting today and will see you."

I haven't seen him, except for a quick "hi," in years. I walked over to the chairs and was almost sitting down when he appeared at the door.

"Come with me to my office," he said.

I followed him nervously down the hall at a brisk pace. I had never seen Dr. Smith in this new office suite, where Drs. Cole and Anderson practiced now that Dr. Smith had retired. The same photos lined the walls and were under his glass desktop. My anxiety rose as Dr. Smith sat me down in a regular chair, not at an exam table. He took my right wrist and felt for my pulse. Immediately, he identified what was going on. "You have atrial fibrillation. It's not a big deal but we need to correct it today."

"What's that?" I asked.

"Atrial fibrillation, or AFib, is an irregular and rapid heart rate or rhythm."

I've never heard of it.

I looked up from my wrist into Dr. Smith's eyes and asked with a shaky voice, "Am I going to die from this?" I had never asked anyone previously if I would die and haven't since. *I don't want to die yet.* I always accepted I might die young, but I never thought it would come so quickly. Picturing a drawn-out death where my heart gradually stopped working effectively, I could prepare everything for my departure, and I was fine with that. *I'm not ready to go so suddenly.*

Reassuringly, Dr. Smith met my eyes and said, "No. This is easily treatable. You need a tune-up for your heart, like a car engine in the shop."

I didn't know what this meant treatment-wise until later, but this analogy made it sound like a common problem. *I can trust Dr. Smith. I'll get better. I'm so glad it's him that's here.*

"I can't treat AFib in my office. You will need to be admitted into the ER." He called ahead and let them know I was on my way and escorted me out of his office. After being in his office for maybe five minutes total, things were moving fast. I had not been to the ER since I fell off my bike when I was seven and now I was almost thirty-one. I started to sweat. *There's going to be so much poking and prodding.*

Before going down to the ER, I called my parents to let them know what was going on. I called home first, but Dad didn't answer, not recognizing the hospital's phone number. I had Mom paged at her office. When she came on the line, I tried not to sound upset, "Everything's okay, and I'm with Dr. Smith, but my heart's sick and I have to go to the ER." Mom had never received a call from me about my heart in my life. I'm sure it was terrifying, but there was some relief knowing I was with Dr. Smith. Mom said they'd meet me in the ER as soon as they could.

The ER

I walked myself slowly down to the ER. Dr. Smith's office was in a building connected to the main hospital and as I walked through the long white halls, I passed by bustling doctors and slow-walking patients. *Don't cry. Think about other things.* Once I arrived, a nurse put me in a wheelchair and wheeled me into a private room. I sat on the white sheet on the bed in my work clothes feeling nervous. *Why are they rushing around? So my heart's beating fast and has been for hours, that's not an emergency.* Nurses hurried me into a hospital gown and hooked me up quickly to an EKG.

A healthy heart beats around 60 to 100 beats per minute, but the numbers on the monitor showed mine at 170. *Dr. Smith was right, not that I doubted him.* To the nurse, I recited my IV mantra of needing the smallest needle possible, a butterfly, and pointed to the spot on my arm with my usable vein, with success on the first try. We shared a grin. My parents arrived shortly afterward. Left alone together for a few minutes, we stared at each other in silence and disbelief, waiting for the doctors to return.

Several minutes later, I grew to hate hearing the machine bleat every time my heart did something irregular. A team of medical students hurried into the room. A young female attending doctor with chin-length black hair and a fleece over her blue scrubs led the team. "You'll have a cardioversion procedure to correct your irregular heartbeat. Cardioversion involves using an electric shock to reset the heart back into its normal rhythm while you are unconscious."

I instantly imagined people on TV getting a shock with large paddles on the chest and people shouting "Clear!" Because cardioversion requires anesthesia, it cannot be performed until six hours after the last meal, the time it takes for the stomach to empty. I had breakfast a few hours earlier so we had a while to wait.

"There is a risk of stroke associated with AFib because it can cause blood clots," the lead doctor told me. "You'll need a transesophageal echocardiogram. Instead of an echo wand that is placed on the chest to see inside the body, a tube to see inside your heart and check for clots will go down your throat while you're asleep."

Fine. I'll be sleeping. Even though the EKG didn't change, I didn't feel panicked as the day went by. *I'm okay. Dr. Smith said I'll get better. The horrible IV's over.*

"We're going to go eat lunch in the cafeteria so you're not tempted," Mom said as she and Dad left the room.

After waiting a few more hours and making nervous small talk with my parents, it was time for the procedures, and the anesthesiologist put me to sleep. When I woke up, I instantly felt the difference in my heartbeat. It was back to normal, and I was a little tired from the anesthesia, which quickly wore off. My throat was sore and the part of my chest where the pads were placed and shocked were red and felt sunburned. I put lotion on the burns, which helped, but there were little twinges of pain throughout the days to come, and the burnt patches itched.

My parents returned to my room in the ER following the procedure and the relief was palpable. The attending doctor came back and said, "You have to spend the night in the hospital." I tried to swallow my fear as the tears poured out of my eyes since no one told me this was going to happen.

"We need to monitor you to make sure that AFib doesn't return and you have no other side effects. There are no rooms upstairs on the hospital floor available, so you'll have to stay the night in the ER in this private room."

My parents tried to comfort me, pointing out I was lucky to have my own room, and they promised to return early in the morning to take me home. *I'm scared. I haven't stayed in the hospital overnight since I was six.* I fell asleep for short periods of time and was frequently woken up by the noises from machines or medical staff passing by. Looking at the clock whenever I felt nervous or lonely, I counted the hours until my parents returned. Focusing on one hour at a time and beginning my count over again when the next hour began got me through the night.

After a restless night, the ER doctor told me I could be discharged. "You need to follow up with your cardiologist with an EKG next week."

"That's easy," I said.

"Upon discharge, you have to take blood thinner pills to prevent the risk of stroke and blood clots for thirty days. The injection you had upon admission to the ER minimized clotting risk, but now the medication will protect you going forward."

I went home with my parents for the weekend to recuperate and mentally process this change in health status. I replayed everything in my mind. *Why did this happen to me? I know I was stressed about the missing luggage, but why would that cause this?*

At my appointment the following week with Dr. Cole, we reviewed everything that happened. "Was it traveler's tummy? Sam researched online and she found one strain of traveler's tummy that can cause AFib," I said.

"There's no way to know right now what caused it. Your stool sample gave no answers," Dr. Cole said. "If AFib happens again, the treatment plan is more cardioversions. There are no studies that reveal long-term consequences to having this procedure multiple times."

I went on with my normal life, hoping it was a one-time occurrence.

It's Back

Four months later, at the end of September 2013, my AFib returned. My gerbil died suddenly on Friday night, causing my heart to start beating irregularly. I paged the cardiology office and Dr. Anderson responded. It had been a long time since Dr. Anderson had cared for me after I opted to see Dr. Cole. Dr. Anderson said in her laid-back style, "The irregular beats could be from the adrenaline from the death and shock. You should wait to see if the irregularity goes away on its own."

I don't know if I believe that, but fine. I don't want to go to the ER over the weekend. It can wait until my physical on Wednesday. I'll have an EKG there to confirm what's going on. Maybe my heart will correct itself. Over the next few days, I learned the longer I was in AFib, the more worn down I felt. *I can't do any unnecessary activities.* My heart beating was impossible to ignore.

I went to work and rested until my office visit.

As expected on Wednesday, my doctor confirmed, "You're in AFib again."

"I knew it," I said sadly.

I was wheeled down to the ER and after check-in, a medical student asked me, "What does AFib feel like?"

Right away, I perked up. *Someone's interested in learning. What a change.* After thinking for a moment about how to respond, I came up with an answer. "It feels like when you have a tired leg muscle that shakes. Instead of your leg shaking, it's your heart shaking." *I hope this helps.*

After our conversation, like the first time I had AFib, I was given a shock to set my heart back into normal rhythm. I woke up feeling better.

"You'll be spending the night upstairs on the cardiac recovery floor," a nurse said.

Oh no. I put on a brave face and smiled at my parents. *I hope this stay's better than last time.*

A few hours later I woke up in my room to a commotion outside at the nurse's desk.

"There's a mouse running around!" a nurse shrieked to the facilities department.

I laughed, hoping to see it myself. The nurse whipped her head around upon hearing my laughter, worried that I might be scared of the mouse.

"Don't worry, it's a small mouse, it can't hurt you," she said as she came to my bedside.

"Oh, I'm not worried. I'm excited and I hope I get to see it!" The nurse left and I looked at the floor but, sadly, never saw the mouse before I went home the following day.

EP Lab

Since AFib recurred, I started seeing a new specialist in the Electrophysiology Lab (EP Lab) at MGH, which specializes in abnormal heart rhythms. It is the clinic to go to for a pacemaker among other things. In October 2013, I had my first EP appointment with Dr. Reid.

Dr. Reid was tall and welcoming. "Hello Emily, I'm happy to meet you," she said in her soothing voice. "I've read about your case and it's unfortunate this is happening, but we're going to work on it together. I'm going to explain everything that's going on with your heart and help you to understand."

She drew some diagrams and explained AFib to me in more detail. "Going forward, if AFib returns, instead of going to the ER for treatment and spending the night in the hospital, you can call me and come to the EP Lab for a cardioversion."

"That's great news. That sounds so much easier."

"We have a procedure room where cardioversions are performed with a team of nurses and doctors who specialize in this procedure. And you'll see me when you come in."

Good, then I'll know someone and won't have to explain my history every time.

"You can go home shortly after the procedure," she said.

The EP Lab might not have had a patient like me, but they seem to know very well how to treat AFib.

"What are all of the possible treatments for AFib? What if cardioversions don't work?"

"Aside from more cardioversions, another treatment option is to start taking medication to try to prevent future AFib episodes. There are only four medications that can be used to treat AFib. However, the medications can also cause lower chamber, ventricular, fibrillation, which can be fatal. To be safe, each one of the four medications, if needed, has to be started in the hospital, under continuous EKG monitoring for three days."

I frowned and looked down. Dr. Reid stopped and let me have a moment, then I looked up at her.

She said, "If the four medications fail, the next treatment step is a cardiac ablation procedure. Cardiac ablation is a procedure performed through the groin area that scars or destroys tissue in the heart that's allowing incorrect electrical signals to cause abnormal heart rhythms. There's an extremely high chance two ablation surgeries will be needed to have long-term success for the treatment of AFib."

Phew, no scars that anyone can see. I nodded.

She continued, "Since we don't know how often you'll have AFib, let's start you on blood thinners. This reduces the risk of stroke, and you won't need transesophageal echoes in the EP Lab. It's not an emergency situation. You don't have to rush to the hospital."

I won't have to cut short a vacation, unless I feel uncomfortable.

"The wait time to administer anesthesia after eating is always six hours. You'll always have time to get to the hospital for treatment and get your personal life in order. You'll need to take off two days from work, one for the procedure and the following day to rest," Dr. Reid said.

At least that part's predictable.

"I'd like to see you back in six months," she said as she finished typing notes on the computer. "That will give us a chance to see if you have another AFib episode."

I'm glad I like her in case this happens a lot.

Hospital Stay

Two months later, the week after Thanksgiving, my heart went into AFib again at the end of a workday.

"Dr. Reid? It's Emily."

"Hi, Emily. How are you?"

"I'm in AFib again, I think."

"Check yourself into the hospital and I'll call in the order to get you started on the first medication."

I hung up the phone and trudged to the subway station.

"We don't have a room available right now," the attendant said. "You'll have to wait and we'll call you when you can come up."

I walked into an empty, dark hallway, past the offices closed for the night. In the hallway, I paced as I called my parents. "I'm in AFib again. Dr. Reid told me to come to the hospital, but they don't have a room ready yet. Can you please bring me some clothes and my toiletries since they won't let me go home to get them myself?"

Tears stung the back of my eyes. *I hate burdening them and needing their help.* We hung up and I sat down to wait.

"I'm sorry for the wait," a nurse said on the phone to me a short while later, and she gave me directions to the hospital floor.

I met the nurse, and she took me to my room where I changed into a hospital gown, was hooked up to an EKG, and lay in the bed. My parents came bustling into the room carrying my overnight bag soon after.

"Nothing can happen tonight. I have to wait for morning," I said as we started unpacking my things together.

"That's all right. You're being monitored, nothing to worry about. We'll see you in the morning. Call us any time," Dad said.

I fell asleep to the erratic bleating of the monitor, which noisily showed me my heart was still irregular.

The next morning, I went to the EP Lab, where I was wheeled to the procedure room. As we went down the halls, the smell of bitter coffee and sweet frosting on pastries made my stomach growl with hunger. After a short wait, I had my cardioversion, woke up in normal rhythm, and was taken back to my room. To test my tolerance for the new medication, sotalol, I stayed in the hospital from Tuesday to Friday.

During my hospital stay, I kept myself busy by ordering my favorite food (spaghetti) from the daily menu and watching TV. My parents came to visit every day and many doctors came in and out to examine me, so I was pretty busy and time flew by. A portable EKG monitor, the size of a medium-sized cell phone, was attached to me 24/7; it prevented me from taking a shower, but I was allowed to walk around and explore my floor. I had a few tests, including an X-ray and an echo, but nothing invasive as I'd feared.

Two days into my hospital stay, I noticed difficulty with my eyesight. Although Dr. Knight's office at the Mass Eye and Ear

Infirmary was in the building next to MGH, I wasn't permitted to be wheeled over for an appointment. "The risk of anything going wrong with your heart while you're at the other hospital is unacceptable," the nurse said.

Something's wrong, but they won't send an eye doctor to me from MGH. I'm not going to sit here quietly and accept doing nothing. My heart's not the only thing that matters. Maybe I'm wrong and my eye's stable, but I don't know. Dr. Knight always tells me to trust my instincts. I called Dr. Knight and she paid me a visit in my hospital room.

When Dr. Knight came in, she was uncharacteristically wearing green scrubs that flapped out behind her like a superhero cape as she briskly came to my bedside. She had her black box with eye lenses to examine me, but no eye-pressure machine. She sat on the edge of my bed and I looked into her portable lenses.

She looked at my eyes and said, "Your eyes are dilated. The pressure's good." It turned out my eyes dilated themselves from being in the hospital, for unknown reasons. "I think they will go back to normal when you are discharged."

Relief washed over me because it was something so simple. I had been correct that my eyes were off, and I was proud of myself for getting an answer.

On Friday, I was discharged from the hospital with no side effects when I returned home. My eyes had returned to normal, and I thought the rest of my body was all right. I was wrong. During my first week at home, I felt awful adjusting to the sotalol, extremely tired and not like myself. Walking to the bus stop or around my small office was exhausting. Since I hadn't been active in the hospital, I hadn't realized the effect the pills were having on me.

Several times throughout the day, I took sotalol. To keep the level of medication high in my bloodstream, the time between pills was short. I could never forget even for a few hours that I was ill, because I had to be on top of the medication timeline just as I had been for the eye drops. After another week or so, I adjusted to the medication and routine. I felt better and more like myself again. Remaining patient, waiting to see if the pills would be effective at keeping AFib away, I tried to forget about my dilemma. At that point, I had had AFib once every three to four months, so I might not know for a while if the pills were doing their job.

New Year, Hospital Stay for Medication Number Two

I rang in the New Year with a cardioversion. My new pet had died and the sadness put me into AFib again. AFib commenced over the holiday weekend and on January 2, 2014, I went in for the first shock of two that week. The medication was not successful at keeping it at bay. The unpredictable nature of my AFib made it impossible to plan ahead. Visits to the EP Lab became a constant part of my routine. It was becoming apparent to me that life with AFib was like riding a roller coaster: fine one moment and in AFib the next, with no way to predict or prevent an episode. *I can't plan my life far in advance. I need to accept that I'm going to miss work and personal events.*

Dr. Reid decided to admit me to the hospital again after my two AFib episodes to start me on amiodarone, the second of the four medications. The hospital stay was similar to the first one, with not much to do except try out the new medication and see if I had any adverse reactions. Growing used to the hospital routine, knowing no unexpected tests involving needles would occur, and having my family visit made me more comfortable. I was no longer afraid to be an inpatient and time went by quickly as I waited and read for three days. When I returned to my condo from the hospital, I was getting ready to shower when I noticed small red dots on my stomach, the size of small pimples but not raised out of the skin. *What the heck is that? I think I got the less than 1 in 10,000 side-effect rash. That's never happened to me before.*

Immediately, I called Dr. Reid and she instructed me to stop taking the medication. Dr. Reid laughed and said, "You aren't making it easy to treat you!" It made me sad to hear the disappointment in her voice when I was feeling so unwell and unable to get better. Despite knowing that it was not my fault, I still felt like I was letting her down. After stopping amiodarone, I resumed taking sotalol, but I didn't have high hopes for its success as it had failed to prevent my previous AFib episodes.

Dr. Reid informed me in her office three days later, "You'll need to have an ablation procedure. We can do it in three to four weeks to prevent further AFib episodes. During the procedure, the doctor will insert catheters through your groin to reach your heart and destroy the tissue causing abnormal heart rhythms from incorrect electrical signals."

I consented to the procedure, which was scheduled for the end of January, about eight months after my first AFib occurrence. Although having a plan was comforting, the frequent hospital visits were taking a toll on my emotional well-being. *Is surgery the right thing to do?*

Dr. Cole reminded me, "Usually once atrial fibrillation becomes more frequent, it's much more difficult to manage with medications alone."

To confirm I had made the right decision to have the ablation, I wanted reassurance from Dr. Smith. Most people need two ablations to be successful in keeping AFib away long-term, so I was prepared for not just one procedure. Dr. Smith and I spoke on the phone.

"I agree you should do this. I want you to do everything you can to combat AFib. Progress is being made in developing treatments for AFib all the time. For some of my patients, I've seen a seventy-five percent success rate with no return of AFib for four to five years. Sometimes it didn't return for ten to twelve years." More often than not, Dr. Smith knew what was best for me, so I committed to having the procedure.

MRI

To prepare for my upcoming ablation, I needed to have an MRI (magnetic resonance imaging) scan to produce a detailed image of my heart. The day before the MRI, I called Dr. Reid to tell her about my latest episode of AFib. I was hesitant to go in for a cardio-version as it might blow my one good vein that I needed for the ablation and MRI.

Dr. Reid said, "You can wait on coming into the lab for a cardioversion because your surgery will correct the rhythm in nine days." It was a relief to have one fewer thing to do and more time at home.

The following day, I had my MRI. The doctors would use the images to create a map of the pathways in my heart. This map would show the specialists during the surgery the tissue to destroy that might be causing AFib. Throughout the MRI, AFib persisted, making it challenging for me to follow the technicians' instructions. They asked me to breathe in different ways and hold my breath to obtain clear images. I nearly had to make myself hyperventilate. It was extremely hard with my breathing already labored from being in AFib since the previous day. The technicians could not understand why it was so difficult for me to breathe in the way they instructed. As I lay in the tube away from everyone, a technician sternly told me over the speaker, "We haven't had many patients in AFib throughout an MRI, but you should be able to do this. Keep trying!"

The technicians continued to forcefully push me to alter my breathing in uncomfortable ways. I tried to stifle my agitation and follow their instructions while quietly kicking my feet. My AFib had been ongoing for so long that I was already exhausted, and their requests only made it worse.

The technicians injected dye into my body during the MRI to create a map for the doctors. When the dye was injected, it felt like I was burning from the inside out. *There was no warning it would feel like this. They only said I might feel some warmth in my groin area. I don't know if I can get through this like other MRIs.* The dye continued to course around my body. *This is total torture. The fire's everywhere.* The burning lasted a minute or two. *Keep staying still, keep holding your breath so that they can get the pictures they need.* I felt warmth in my groin. *I think I peed my pants. One ... two ... three ... one ... two—* One of these times it will be over.

The pounding in my chest from AFib and exhaustion didn't lessen over the days in advance of the ablation. Dr. Reid said on the phone, "Unless you really need to, you don't have to come in for a cardioversion. Just know you will become more tired and worn down if you don't." I decided I needed to go in. I went in for my sixth cardioversion prior to the surgery, following the MRI.

Feelings before the Ablation

After my cardioversion, I had more energy. I walked to the bus stop without feeling winded and was able to stay awake after work for longer than the week previously. Unfortunately, feeling better quickly faded. My hopes for a positive outcome of the surgery were low, and I knew there was a possibility that I might need a second ablation.

I tried to stay outwardly positive to keep my family's and my own spirits up, if only temporarily. For the next week, I lost interest in my favorite things, such as reading and television. Instead, I spent most of my time on the couch, waiting for the surgery. Four days after my last episode, I went into AFib again. I didn't have another cardioversion and waited for the surgery two days later.

First Ablation

Early in the morning of January 30, 2014, I had the ablation. The procedure took place in the EP Lab. Whereas my cardioversions had been done in the hall behind a white curtain, for the ablation

I was wheeled through two swinging brown doors into a private sterile room. Dr. Reid stayed with me until I fell asleep.

During the surgery, the surgeon used two different techniques to modify the tissues and electrical pathways that were sending the imperfect signals into my heart to stop future episodes of AFib from happening. He used extreme cold (freezing cryoablation) and heat (radiofrequency energy) through catheters and wire electrodes.

When I woke up in the recovery room I was no longer in AFib, but there were still two catheters in my groin area. I needed to remain lying flat for six hours. During that time, I drifted in and out of consciousness. The procedure to remove the catheters was especially vivid. A nurse came over and told me they would be pulling them out, one at a time. I tried to sleep through the worst of it. After the removal, when I woke up a few seconds later, a nurse was standing up and pressing extremely hard with both of her hands interlocked on one side of my groin to stop the bleeding from the incisions. In ablations, stitches are not used to close the wounds and the body has to naturally heal itself because the incisions are not deep. There was sharp pain from the pressure and I had to keep myself from pushing her hands off of me in defense. It was like a brick was being pressed onto my leg in a sensitive spot and I felt a swollen mound underneath her fingers. I stared at the wall while this was happening so I wouldn't see anything. Eventually, the bleeding ended and the nurse stopped pressing so hard.

A couple of minutes later, when I woke up again, I saw the nurse at the end of my bed writing something down on my chart. I felt a warm trickle near my groin. Although I was weak and my voice was quiet from the soreness of the transesophageal echo, I whispered, "I'm leaking" and the nurse heard me. She came over and lifted my gown and applied pressure again to the bleeding wounds. I fell back asleep and after a while it was time to move to my recovery room for the night.

In my bed, I was wheeled up to the recovery floor because I needed to lie flat. When my parents and I arrived in my room, I was moved around so that a large sheet could be placed under my body. *What's happening?* The nurses fussed around, straightening the sheet out along the length of my body. I was told I would be lifted into the air and over to the bed in a sling. *I feel like a dolphin being rescued and returned to the sea.* I crossed my arms over my chest, and the machine lifted me up. I rose higher and higher away from everyone. The sling pushed my arms against the center of my body and squished my legs. *Ow, that hurts my incisions.* The bleeding risk meant I couldn't move, and it was not a good idea to get fidgety so high up, so I kept my eyes open and stared at the ceiling. *I hope this ends soon. It feels like a Ferris wheel and I hate amusement park rides.* The large sheet underneath me was removed as I was lowered onto the bed. Relieved to no longer be flying, I took in my surroundings and saw a normal hospital room with an adjustable bed, a night table, a TV hanging in front of me, and a whiteboard displaying the date and my nurses' and doctors' names. I had a roommate behind a curtain on the window side of the room, so I couldn't see any views except into the hallway across from the nurse's station.

I still needed to lie flat in the bed for a while longer, and I talked with my parents prior to their return home in the evening. Keeping my eyes closed, I listened to Mom and Dad tell me stories about the neighborhood pets and people as entertainment. Before going home for the night, trying to reassure me, Dad said, "No more negative thoughts, just positive thoughts now."

Three hours later I could get up and sit in a chair. I was about to go to the restroom when my nurse spoke to me. She warned me, "When you pee for the first time it might burn, and it also might be red-colored from the iodine."

I went to the bathroom and looked in the bowl. *There's a red sea! Calm down, she told you this would happen. It's not unexpected blood.* I positioned my hospital gown to cover my incisions so I didn't have to look at them. The nurse stayed outside the door while I was in the restroom, reassuring me. After that, I went back to bed and mostly slept, as I was not feeling up to doing much.

Collapsed Lung

The next morning I woke up groggy, then quickly fully alert. I saw a thin, tall man with black hair in a crew cut, standing up perfectly straight, writing notes on my chart. I could tell he was a medical student. He turned to me and giddily said, "Did you hear about what went wrong during the procedure?" There is nothing worse than that to hear after waking up from any surgery. I was incensed and alone with the student as he gave me the bad news, which he appeared excited about. "One of your lungs collapsed during the surgery."

Dr. Reid told me that was a risk. I expected something much worse after his comment. I feel fine. I'll ask her if I should be concerned. Fuming about the student's poor bedside manner and how he had no concept of how poorly he had acted, I focused on my anger at him rather than my lung.

Dr. Reid and the surgeon came to visit me a short while later. Dr. Reid patiently told me, "Your lung might or might not heal itself; time will tell. Everything else went well although your heart was surgically challenging."

The surgeon then chipped in, "The procedure took longer than expected. Nevertheless, I figured it out and did what had to be done." Both Dr. Reid and the surgeon agreed I could be discharged that day. I then ranted about the medical student, whom she agreed to speak with about his technique for delivering information to patients. I calmed down and focused on getting ready to go home.

After two more hours in my hospital room, I was ready to be discharged. I experienced pain in my thighs during the recovery week at my parents' house. The cold energy dispersed during the ablation caused the pain. I pressed on my legs during the discomfort and waited it out, as there was nothing I could do to stop it. The pain came in random bursts, so medication was not effective in providing relief. I tried to distract myself by watching television, but there were times when I just had to wait until the hurt subsided.

I could not do anything to strengthen or repair my collapsed lung either. I was able to manage it, with the exception of two noticeable things: I could not take a full, deep breath, which meant that my breath would cut short and that I could not complete a full yawn, and my sneezes were smaller. Additionally, I developed a hiccup-like gasp that happened randomly and unconsciously. My breath sort of hiccupped and then sucked in for a second. Sometimes it happened a few times throughout the day and sometimes it happened a small number of times throughout an hour. After a couple of days, I could tell that my lung was no longer collapsed. I was able to take deeper breaths. The hiccup-like breathing was happening less frequently, but even years later, I still experience it on occasion without knowing why, even though my lung has corrected itself.

During my recovery week, I settled into a routine at my parents' house. Listening to the lyrics in the chorus of Katy Perry's song "Roar" helped me to feel better and stronger again. I wanted to be as strong as I had been prior to AFib, and the lyrics fit that theme. It usually took me three or four days to get back to my pre-cardioversion strength, and I anticipated a similar recovery pattern after the ablation. This recovery was roughly the same as with a cardioversion, merely a couple of days longer. My breathing was a bit more labored when walking or going up the stairs, and I needed to build my stamina back up.

To regain my strength, I went on daily neighborhood walks with Dad. We developed this routine after cardioversions and continued it after the ablation. During our walks, we saw the neighborhood dogs and cats, which I enjoyed a great deal. The daily walks helped me to be aware of my progress, and each day, I was able to walk further and become stronger.

Bandage Removal

Two days after discharge from the hospital, I needed to do something I dreaded: removing the bandages from my groin. *The incisions will open. I'm going to bleed. There are no stitches holding me together. I'll slowly peel them off in the shower.* I was crying out of fear and needed moral support in the room.

Sam had come home for my surgery to be with me. She had missed a lot of my illnesses throughout the years and all of the cardioversion procedures because she went to school out of state. Usually, I couldn't bring myself to admit to her how I was really feeling. During this recovery, she had been a great help and I confided my true feelings to her. She stood in the room with me for the removal, "You can do it. It'll be over soon."

I cried and peeled the clear bandages off. She held a garbage can for me outside of the shower curtain and I passed the used bandages into it. I stopped crying once they were gone. To my immense relief, the bandages came off without any unexpected bleeding.

After I dressed, I joined my family to watch a movie. During the movie, my AFib returned. *I'm going to have to have surgery again.* The beats felt gigantic. *This feels like when people say their heart beat out of their chest. Being so upset from taking off the bandages caused it.* Fortunately, the horrible beating stopped on its own and I never felt such deep beating again. Sadly, the shallower normal AFib I usually experienced returned shortly after the bandage removal episode.

New Month, New AFib Medication

Following my first ablation, my doctors warned me that my sensitivity to irregular heartbeats would dissipate after each one. Prior to the surgery, I could always pinpoint, to the minute, when a new episode of AFib began. This is not the case for many people, who either can't feel it as strongly or don't notice it at all. The younger doctors in the EP Lab found it amusing that I could say to the minute when AFib started, as they were not used to someone being so cognizant of their body.

After this first surgery, I found I could still feel AFib as strongly as I had prior to the ablation, but I became obsessed with regularly checking my pulse in my neck to count my heartbeats per minute to confirm whether or not I was in AFib. When I called Dr. Reid to tell her I was in AFib again early in the week after the ablation, she said, "It's unfortunate it is so soon after the procedure; however, it is not unexpected. After the ablation, the arrhythmia may sometimes get worse before it gets better." We decided to give my heart time to see if it would settle on its own. It did, but AFib quickly returned again.

In February, two weeks after the procedure, I went into the lab twice for cardioversions. At the end of the second week after the ablation, I was admitted into the hospital for the initiation of the third AFib medication. During this hospital stay, a snowstorm blew in and my parents couldn't come to visit me right away. *It's my first cardioversion without them. It's going to be hard, but I won't have to pretend I'm fine or make jokes when I feel so tired.* After the cardioversion in the EP Lab, I was taken up to my room on the hospital floor to be monitored while starting the new medication.

My parents came to visit me the following day and Mom brought me a slice of cake from the cafeteria to celebrate Valentine's Day. It was vanilla cake with white frosting and a plastic pink and red heart topper. Savoring the sugary frosting made my day much better, and I decorated my wall with the tiny cake topper.

To keep busy during my hospital stay, I read books and often walked down the hall to sit beside a fish tank. Multicolored tropical fish of all sizes and shapes swam around white sand, coral, and plants waving in the bubbles. Next to the tank, through the doors, was a neonatal (infant) unit, and the sharp wailing of the babies could be heard. While looking at the fish, I reminded myself, *stay strong, don't cry like the babies.* When I looked at the fish, I imagined being free to explore once I regained the ability to travel again. *You only have a few more days to get through. You'll go home soon. It could be much worse.*

The medication I started in the hospital was called flecainide. When I left the hospital and went back to my condo and work, my quality of life vanished. This medicine made me so tired that I napped every day and I could no longer work full-time. Dr. Reid wrote to my manager at work to explain my absence, "Emily is affected physically by the recent procedure, the recurrent atrial fibrillation, and the visits to the hospital. Although she maintains a positive attitude, she needs to remain at home to rest. I have recommended she returns to a part-time duty of four hours per day until April 30. ... This is the period that we may still expect recurrences of the arrhythmia and need for hospital visits."

This is so embarrassing. I hate telling my manager this private stuff. I guess I have to so she can understand. I don't like missing so much work. I do feel crummy though. I can't work a full day. During this time, I often felt alone with few people to talk to and little energy to interact with others. To try to take some advantage of my time out of the office and not feel completely isolated, I ate lunch specials at restaurants on my way home to make part of the day feel worthwhile. I'd often eat at a Thai restaurant that was usually pretty empty as I'd arrive around 1:30. Walking into the restaurant, I was hit with the aromas of spicy foods people ordered. I looked at their plates to see what they were eating as I walked slowly to my table past the peach-colored walls. The smells of satay skewers, dumplings, and warm soup filled the air. My stomach turned in hunger. I sat down at my table and savored my usual go-to lunch special of tofu pad thai, dumplings, and tom yum soup. I'd eat slower than usual to prolong my time at the

restaurant. *Pretend you're on vacation. I'm eating in an exotic land.*
I watched the people passing by outside and imagined a life where
I'd feel healthy enough to return to work full-time again and travel.
After I finished, I'd walk home exhausted and lonely, with only my
television for entertainment.

AFib Lifestyle Changes

During this time, I required several cardioversions and went to the
hospital every couple of days for the procedure. Over the course
of six months, I had more than thirty episodes that needed treatment. AFib would start at unpredictable times, and I was unable
to determine what triggered each episode, nor could the doctors.
One time I was in the line at the post office, another it was excitement from getting a new gerbil, once it was anger when a manager
was stern with me at work, another time I was simply standing in
the shower washing my hair. I learned to control my emotions, as
stress and excitement seemed to trigger it.

I easily went through the motions of my AFib routine without thinking about it. Each day followed the same monotonous
pattern. If my heart didn't start beating irregularly during the day,
I would inevitably wake up in the night to the irregular beating of
my heart. *I can't sleep with this pounding.* The beating always felt
stronger when I lay on my side or back and sitting or standing up
made it less noticeable.

When Dr. Reid returned my early morning call, I caught her
up on when AFib had begun.

"Hello?" I said into my phone when she called me back.

"It started again," I said. Hanging up after our conversation,
I knew who I needed to call next.

"Hi Mom," I said on the phone. "I'm in AFib again. We're
spending the day in the hospital."

"Okay. When should we get there?" she said.

"I don't know, the nurse hasn't called me back yet. I'll text you."

The hours leading up to going to the hospital were a time of freedom before the anxiety of the hospital visit took over and things were out of my control. *Do some chores now. I still feel medium good and I'll feel worse later after the shock.* To keep busy and keep my hunger away I began preparing food for the next few days. *Cooking will distract me and I won't feel hungry. When it gets to be too much and I'm tired, I'll stop and rest.*

A few hours after our initial call, Dr. Reid or a nurse called me from the lab to schedule a cardioversion. Once my appointment was confirmed, I emailed my manager at work to inform her that I would be out of work for the next two days. My medical problems were not met with compassion in my demanding office. As the episodes became more frequent, I missed a significant amount of work, needing to take off the procedure day and the following day to rest at home. On one occasion, I called to tell my boss about my upcoming absence and she said, "You can no longer have unpredictable absences."

That's a ludicrous and unfair thing to say to anyone! She's blaming me for something I can't control. I can't make this better!

Some days when I had a particularly arduous time physically and emotionally, feeling worn down and sad, I didn't eat even if I wasn't in AFib. *AFib might come at any moment and I don't want to wait six hours for help.*

Sometimes I was at work when AFib began and I scheduled a cardioversion several hours later, trying to miss as little work as possible. I went about my workday when I could and working part-time helped so I could have a cardioversion after work if I felt I could wait.

Once the procedure was scheduled, I typically left my office or my home and rode the subway to the hospital. I met my parents prior to entering the lab in the hospital hallway. Walking by the bakery right outside the lab, I saw and smelled all the food I couldn't eat behind glass cabinets. *Look at all the delicious frosting. Ooh, big chocolate chip cookies and fruit.* I smelled freshly brewed coffee and heard the machines grinding away making everyone's drinks.

"Dad, guess which one I'll order?"

"That cookie." He'd point.

"I want frosting, this time, so I'll get that cake slice."

Entering the EP Lab, I checked in at the main desk and the staff printed me a hospital identification bracelet to wear. *I hate these bracelets. Everyone can see now that I'm the sick one. What must they imagine is wrong with me?* Until the procedure, I fiddled with my bracelet and when it was loose enough I slipped it on and off. "Look, I don't have a bracelet on. I can go home now," I said to my parents. *We can escape all this.*

In the L-shaped waiting room, I chose my seat carefully. I had two options: sit by the door to the hallway across from the reception desk and watch doctors come in and out of the room, hidden from the procedure room entrance, or sit on the long side of the "L" with the procedure and exam room entrances across from each other and watch nurses call patients in for their appointments. Sometimes I preferred to hide from the nurses on the far side, while at other times I paced in front of my seated parents, feeling anxious to get the IV over with and feel better.

I said, "I want to go home" and they laughed uncomfortably. *I want to get better and stop feeling this way, but I don't really want to go through the cardioversion.*

"You can go home in an hour or two," Dad said. My parents made their own jokes to mask their worry, but they were concerned. *They're so worried. Pretend everything's all right.* "Look at this dress. It's so ugly," I said pointing to a photo in a magazine.

"I agree, but what do you think of this one?" Mom said.

"I vote for the other dress."

After the wait, a nurse called me back into the lab. I quickly stood up and handed Mom my phone and valuables and followed the nurse. Once we went a couple of short steps into the procedure room, she told me to go into the restroom and put on a hospital gown. In the restroom, I checked my pulse one last time. *I hope I'm in AFib. I don't want to be embarrassed, if I'm wrong.* I was always in AFib, never mistaken.

After I left the restroom, they took me to an open room with two beds with a curtain between them. The shelves behind the beds were full of machines and tubing waiting for the patients. At times another patient, usually elderly, was in the other bed. *I'm always the youngest here!*

More often than not, I was alone in the room. The black railings of the bed were lowered for me and I'd sit on the white sheet. After taking off my shoes, I'd lie on the bed and a nurse hooked me up to an EKG. My heartbeat clocked in around 156 to 170 beats per minute. *Stupid machine. It's so loud every time my heart beats incorrectly. At least I was right that I'm sick.* In the beginning of my AFib episodes, Dad came with me inside the lab and sat with me while we waited for the procedure to start.

"Use the butterfly needle and this vein," I said confidently to the anesthesiologist. *I'm so used to seeing needles in my body now, I don't have to look away anymore. It's probably because I've done this so many times.* "I ate over six hours ago and I took my blood thinner medication."

The next step to prepare for the cardioversion was placing the two large orange cardioversion pads on my body, one on the center of my chest and one on my back. After that, I waited in the bed for Dr. Reid and the other doctors to arrive, which could take a while. When Dr. Reid arrived at my bedside, it signaled procedure time and I would soon be going to sleep. "How are you doing, Emily? Do you have any questions?" Other doctors returned to my bedside and gathered around the foot of my bed to review the upcoming procedure. The team called this a "time out." All action stopped around me while my allergies, anesthesia, and procedure were reviewed.

They know all about me. I'll be fine. It's nice and calm now.

The anesthesiologist injected medication into my IV to put me to sleep. "It tastes sour in the back of my throat," I said to the anesthesiologist as it coursed through my veins.

"Not many people report that, but it's normal."

As I drifted off, I looked at Dr. Reid at the foot of my bed. *She'll take excellent care of me. She's always here. I trust her and her judgment.* Sometimes it felt like I could keep myself awake and I continued to look at Dr. Reid, but most times I wanted to feel better and let the medicine take over. I'd feel the propofol anesthesia working when I felt almost dizzy, with my head starting to spin. Knowing it was time to let it work, I'd put my head down on the pillow, close my eyes and let go.

Once I was asleep, the doctors shocked my heart back into normal rhythm. I woke up a short while later and quickly became fully alert after the anesthesia. *My heart's back in normal rhythm. There's no pounding in my chest.* Confirming what I felt, I looked at the EKG monitor and saw a normal heart rate.

"We were able to shock you once and your heart reset," the nurse said. Every so often I'd see Dr. Reid again when I woke up, but most of the time, I did not.

After getting dressed, I signed the discharge paperwork and went back out into the waiting room to meet my parents.

"Time to eat. What do you want?" Dad said.

"Chicken salad." Sometimes we went to the cafeteria and I'd eat the food I joked about wanting earlier, and other times I went directly home. Since I no longer stayed in the hospital overnight after cardioversions, initially I would go to my parents' house after the procedure so they could help me during recovery. At times, I was too tired to care for myself or prepare my own food, so going to their house was easier and they felt reassured watching over me. Later, as the AFib incidents became more routine, I simply returned to my condo and took care of myself. I prepared food in bulk so it was ready when I wasn't up for cooking. As I've never enjoyed cooking, I made myself a week's worth of pasta with butter and garlic on it.

Back at home, I applied lotion to the sunburned areas where the pads had been and waited for the strange tingles and twinges to stop. After eating, I either took a nap or watched TV, taking it easy.

The recovery process usually took one day, but sometimes I needed an extra day or two. If I didn't receive a cardioversion soon after the AFib episode, the next day I woke up feeling crummy. *My breathing's labored. I need more air to feel like I've filled my lungs.* Sometimes, I experienced an overall sense of exhaustion. Following cardioversions, even climbing two or three steps to enter the house felt like a demanding task that couldn't be avoided, no matter how much I wanted to.

During the height of my AFib episodes, it became normal to feel tired, look pale, and not want to do much. The steam and warmth in the shower made it difficult for me to breathe, so I lowered the water temperature. I stopped preparing my own lunch when I worked full days and instead opted to eat out since it required less effort than cooking.

I can't remember a life before AFib. I know time's passing because the pills in the bottle are dwindling, but every day feels the same. I can't plan anything more than a day in advance. I never know when I'll be at the hospital. But it's probably very soon. There were bad days when I felt discouraged and irritated: the ups-and-downs of chronic illness. *I'm so tired of being tired. Treatment isn't pointless, though. I can be fixed for a day or two and go back to my old life routines.*

I never gave up altogether trying to take part in normal activities. *Doing anything is still something.* I didn't have the stamina to take care of most of my household chores, like vacuuming. *Vacuum one room instead of three. Clean one counter today.* Instead of going to a restaurant downtown with a friend I suggested a restaurant near my office or home so I wouldn't have to be out as long.

I can't really talk about this with my friends or people at work. I know there's only so much negative news someone can listen to. I know they'd be sympathetic and supportive but I have nothing positive to say, so I'll keep to myself. I enjoyed seeing Dr. Reid and the nurses in the office because they could understand what was going on with me and I had someone I could talk to about what was happening. The office staff made jokes when they'd see me in the waiting room just about every week saying "Not again" or "You again, what are you doing here?" I'd laugh as we all recognized I had no control of the situation.

Why Now?

Why is this happening to me? I was stable from six to almost thirty-one. Why am I having so many irregular heartbeat episodes?

I asked Dr. Cole at one of my checkups why this was occurring. She theorized, "For the six years before your first surgery when the blood was regurgitating instead of circulating around your body, your left atrium grew larger because some of the blood was pushed backward into it with every heartbeat." She paused so I could process this information and then continued, "The left atrium continued to slowly enlarge over the years and the enlargement or the leaking of the mitral valve could be what triggered AFib. The electrical pathways behave incorrectly and cause AFib."

Treatment decisions made when I was younger, when my first surgery was postponed until age six, were now affecting me all these years later. *There's no one older to compare me to, to learn how to treat me. There's no one to study to see what outcomes they had.* Surgeons now perform surgery on ALCAPA patients in infancy and mitral valve rings are no longer used. *At least Dr. Cole has somewhat of a possible reason for why this is happening.*

I reminded myself, *this won't be forever. If you give up because of this, you can't fight future problems.* If the AFib couldn't be corrected with each episode or if I had pain that lingered for months I'm not sure I could have seen the other side and stayed positive. *Live with the hand you're dealt. Something's always gonna change. Don't feel defeated.*

AFib Medications

The AFib pill, flecainide, is awful. Everything exhausted me and I couldn't walk at my normal pace. *It's not even working well. My heart's moving so fast, but I'm a snail on the outside. I can stay positive for cardioversions, but this medicine makes me so down and angry.*

On my way to work one morning, I struggled to climb the steep stairs at the subway station exit. The stairs at this station were always strenuous for me and I was noticeably slower than usual. As a distraction from the incline as I went up the stairs I was looking down at my phone, texting with Sam, but that was not what was slowing me down; it was the annoying medicine.

The station was crowded and I kept to the right as I slogged up the staircase, along the wall, to keep out of the way of commuters. A woman screamed at me, "Get off the damn phone and hurry up!" She hurried by me and disappeared.

I can't keep up with her. I wish I could scream at her, "The phone has nothing to do with it. It's my heart!" There wasn't an escalator I could take instead, and I couldn't make my body move faster. *I know it's commuting time and everyone's in their own world, but she had no idea what's slowing me down. She should've been more considerate.* I stewed about it for days.

Instead of screaming at someone on the subway with my frustration, I began calling my medication "fuckinide" because I hated what it was doing to me. I called Dr. Reid in March, one month after starting to take flecainide, and said firmly but weakly, "I won't wait until our next checkup at the end of April to make a change. I can't stand this medicine and I don't want to take it anymore!" In my head I sounded assertive, but I might actually have been subdued because I was exhausted and more quiet than usual; she understood and agreed to let me take the fourth and last possible medication.

Propafenone was prescribed, and it proved effective for a period of time. By May, I was able to return to full-time work after four months of part-time work, and my limited energy returned. If I felt symptoms of AFib, I could take more doses of propafenone and cardioversions were not always necessary. This was an improvement since my heart had never reverted to a normal rhythm on its own without cardioversions. I started experiencing minor episodes of atrial flutter, a similar abnormal heart rhythm to AFib, causing rapid heartbeats. Cardioversions are not effective for atrial flutter as they treat specific rhythms. When I felt flutter, I took an extra propafenone pill and it made atrial flutter episodes disappear and sometimes they resolved on their own without pills.

After work, I went straight home in order to take my blood thinner medication at the same time every night and ate a large dinner, an obligation for the medication to work properly and not cause side effects. I took propafenone at the appointed times, four times a day, to keep my levels high to keep AFib away. This worked for a while, and I planned a vacation with Sam to France in May.

France

In mid-May, ahead of going to France, some AFib returned, as did my need for cardioversions. I began to walk slowly again, though I never felt as poorly as I had on flecainide. At an appointment with Dr. Reid, as she sat next to me at her desk, she said, "I am concerned about the progression of your AFib episodes. The medication was controlling your heart more effectively a few weeks ago, but now is no longer as successful."

A lump rose in my throat and I tried not to cry. I desperately wanted to go to France and tried to bargain with Dr. Reid. "I'll go back on flecainide if I have to," I said, discouraged. *My trip to DC was already postponed because of AFib. I don't want to cancel any more vacations.*

Dr. Reid thought for a moment since she knew I needed this trip to improve my morale. "Instead of postponing your vacation, let's try higher doses of propafenone. You can get a cardioversion in France if needed. The ablation procedure was invented there." I was surprised to hear this and glad to have a solution. I also had local friends who could help translate at the hospital if needed and I'd be with Sam.

Dr. Reid's such a good doctor. She cares about my quality of life. When I asked her about coming home early from France if AFib returned and I didn't want to go to the hospital there, she answered, "You can wait for as long as you tolerate it, but you have to be honest with yourself. You can certainly wait until you come back."

She then asked gently, "Would you consider, after you come back, discussing another ablation?" I appreciated how she handled the delicate topic since she knew I didn't want a second one because the outcomes of the first had not been great.

"Yes, I will," I tentatively agreed. *She conceded to things for me, so I can too. But I'll decide after I'm back from France.*

On May 22nd, I had my final appointment in the EP Lab before leaving for France. As a precaution, I had scheduled a cardioversion for the last possible day before my trip. My AFib was not strong that day and I didn't qualify for a cardioversion. Even if I'd had a cardioversion, there was no guarantee that I would have stayed in normal rhythm throughout the night or beyond. At that point, my cardioversions had not provided me more than a couple of hours of relief. I understood the risks and what I was getting into by going away, but I also understood it might be my last trip for a while because another surgery was looming.

Going to France in my weakened state taught me about my limitations during my AFib reoccurrences. Napping throughout the day on park benches, I was slow and had little energy. I shopped for clothes with Sam while taking frequent rests on changing room chairs. The entire time, I was in atrial flutter that never corrected itself. I avoided tackling any stairs or hills that weren't compulsory and didn't participate in activities that I hadn't planned ahead of time. Some attractions were impossible for me to visit, so Sam took pictures to show me what I had missed and brought me food that I couldn't walk to get myself, such as pastries from our favorite bakery. I savored their sweet fruit fillings and chocolate toppings. Unable to walk around museums or through long street markets, this was not an enjoyable quality of life. I decided to have the surgery when I returned.

Back in Boston, I didn't feel much like myself, markedly tired and worn down from the AFib and the emotions caused by constant abnormal heart rhythms. In mid-June, two weeks after my return, I saw Dr. Reid for a checkup. I had been looking forward to telling her about France, but the appointment didn't go as expected. My heart rate was high and she confirmed, "You should have the second ablation surgery as soon as possible." A bit surprised, since she never acted like anything was urgent, I had assumed the second surgery would be like the first ablation, where I could have cardioversions as needed awaiting the scheduled surgery. Instead, Dr. Reid said, "Your pulse is too high to continue on the cardioversion routine, and it's not effective given the AFib keeps returning."

I meekly asked, "What are the next steps if the second ablation fails?"

"Instead of having a third ablation surgery, you will have to think about a pacemaker as a more permanent solution."

I tried not to worry over this news and scheduled my second ablation for July 3, 2014, weeks before my thirty-second birthday. Dad told me to hope for the best and expect the worst, as my expectations and spirits were low.

Round Two

Although the second ablation surgery was merely five months after the first, it was a vastly improved experience. During the MRI and the surgery, I wasn't in AFib, and I insisted that the catheters be removed while I was still asleep. When the machine lifted me into my bed, I was accustomed to it and wasn't as nervous as before. Additionally, when I noticed that my urine was red, I knew what it was.

On the night of the ablation, a thunderstorm echoed through the sky, keeping me awake. I didn't feel like watching television, so I gazed at the reflection of the lightning flashing across the sky in the window next to my roommate's bed. I could also hear nearby July 4th fireworks, which were entertaining to listen to from my bed. Occasionally, I could see the fireworks' reflections bursting on the television.

The day following the procedure, I did not have a collapsed lung, unlike the first time. I went to my parents' home and worked on recovering for the week. Except for a few flutters, I did not have any irregular heartbeats. Dad and I went on daily walks throughout the neighborhood.

I resumed working full-time on July 14th. Remaining on blood thinners for a while was frustrating. I ate at the same time every night when I took the medication and the heavy blood loss from small cuts was annoying. Dr. Reid gradually reduced my propafenone dosage as my heart continued to stabilize. After the second surgery, I experienced AFib only one evening in July, and an additional propafenone pill made it disappear the following morning. I still occasionally felt flutters, but I was generally doing well.

Vacation with Mabel

Feeling stronger after the ablation, I decided it was time to to get together with Mabel. We went to Martha's Vineyard for a three-day summer vacation. We walked along the manicured lawns and admired the pretty flowers while talking about TV shows and medical updates.

"Do you have any new scars?" Mabel said.

"Yeah, in my groin area. They're hard to see," I said.

"That's too bad, but I'm glad you're better now."

"It's worth it not to have to have any more IVs or Holter monitors. That's for sure."

"Ick, the worst," she agreed. "Did the doctor say what'll happen if this ablation doesn't work?"

"Yeah, I'd have to get a pacemaker, like you."

Mabel was silent for a moment. "It's not that big of a deal. It can be annoying, but maybe it's better than what you've been dealing with."

A few weeks later, Mabel called to let me know her friend, who had the same heart condition she has, passed away suddenly from a stroke.

"I don't think suddenly dying is a huge risk for either of us," I said on the phone with Mabel. "But it could happen to anyone and we've always known it's a possibility."

"I think we have a different level of anxiety about this," Mabel said tentatively. "Anyone could have a freak accident or be hit by a car. But I know multiple people our age who have died from their conditions. I spoke to my doctor about what happened. He said we could consider trying a blood thinner to reduce the risk of stroke."

"I've taken that medication, and it's awful! Every time I had a cardioversion I was on it for thirty days," I said. "Tiny cuts bled a lot, I gained weight, and I had a heavy period for weeks. It was terrible. I don't think you should take it unless you have no other options. Your doctor might not have considered these side effects when he told you about the pill."

I don't want to scare her, but she has to know the realities of living with this medication.

Mabel paused, and I could hear her crack her knuckles on the phone. "This is super helpful. I'm gonna have another conversation with my doctor about it."

A week later, the phone rang and I cheerily answered, "Hi, Mabel."

"Hi," came Mabel's familiar voice.

"How's it going?"

"Fine," she said. "I had my cardio appointment and we decided that pill wasn't necessary for me. A daily baby aspirin is a better place to start for now."

"That's good. Was it hard to bring it up with your doctor?"

"It wasn't hard at all," Mabel replied. "I told him about your negative experience and he agrees that I don't need to jump to that level of medication."

"What about the chance of dying? Did that come up?"

"A little … but I really talk more about that with you."

"Me too. I can't talk about that with my family. Oh, by the way, I had an echo and the person really hurt me. Does it hurt you too, so much, when the wand digs into your stomach to see your heart?"

Mabel sighed. "Yes. We have to grin and bear it sometimes since we don't have a choice."

"I just fake-smile and grit my teeth, staring at the ceiling."

"Did you tell your parents?" she asked.

"No, they won't understand and I have to get the test done. I don't want to go back."

UAE and the Gym

I had one lone incident of AFib in February 2015, seven months after the second ablation. The incident resolved on its own, which was a relief since I was going on vacation a few days later. I visited the United Arab Emirates (UAE) for two weeks, fulfilling a long-time desire. I seized the opportunity to fully explore the country and immersed myself in local culture. I attended an Emirati dinner that was a bridge between cultures, where I learned about customs and enjoyed saffron rice, chickpeas, and spicy mixed vegetables, but the highlight was the donuts drenched in date syrup. Visiting an island where African animals had been imported, I went on a safari. I greatly enjoyed seeing cheetahs and rock hyraxes, small gray animals that look like rodents and live in rocks, but are most closely related to elephants.

One of the most fascinating experiences I had in the UAE was attending a camel race. Instead of jockeys, little robots that sit on top of saddles control the camels. The owners of the camels employ people who remotely control the jockeys via radio transmitter to make the camels run faster. I had the unique opportunity to ride alongside the camels in the media van, which transmits a live radio broadcast. As the camels raced around the track multiple times, I could see the little robots in action, and the spit flying off the camels' cheeks.

I had a great time there and felt my life was getting back on track after the difficult year I had been through. When I returned to Boston, I decided it was time to join a gym for the first time in my life since Dr. Cole had approved it. A major difference between Dr. Cole and Dr. Smith is that Dr. Cole is a proponent of exercise. Dr. Smith never pushed me to try new things or suggested physical activity. His answer to most new activities I wanted to try was no. In college, I asked, "Can I go indoor rock climbing and quit if it's too hard?" Of course, he said no. He wanted me to sit and rest and never exert or push myself, but Dr. Cole has a different perspective.

It took me years to feel brave and strong enough to take her exercise advice to heart, and I was finally ready. This new openness to activity didn't mean my abilities somehow changed overnight and I would be physically capable of more or even coordinated enough to succeed. But I wanted to challenge myself and prove I could become stronger. *I can always stop if it's too much.*

After work, I began going to a gym in my neighborhood and started taking group fitness classes like Zumba and aerobics, but they were tough. I stood in the back, not looking at myself in the mirror, trying to keep up with all the moves the teacher demonstrated. *I'm tired and I can't keep up. This is embarrassing.* I stopped attending the classes. I tried using the machines, but I didn't know how to use any of them; I'd only walked on a treadmill a couple of times at hotels previously.

My gym membership came with a free personal training session, and I found I liked it very much. The trainer taught me how to use the machines and we discovered that I enjoyed kickboxing. I hadn't boxed since I was a child and hit my punching bag in my basement at home to take out my anger after the first surgery. Taking out some of my built-up aggression about AFib helped me become stronger at the same time. The trainer tailored the workouts to my ability and went at my pace. I kicked and punched her pads directly in a competitive way, keeping me motivated to progress. I never did more than what I assumed I could do and stuck to a comfortable level of activity that didn't raise my heart rate much. When I was out of breath or my heart rate rose, I stopped to rest. *Don't go too far.* I merely tried to become stronger and more confident in the strength I did have.

One Year AFib Free

In July 2015, before I turned thirty-three, I had a party at home with my parents to commemorate one year without AFib. We celebrated a successful year; I had been to the UAE, gone to the gym, trained with a personal trainer, and learned how to box. Feeling stronger than I had in a long, long time, I had been more physically active than I could remember in the past. I gorged on a box of cookies from my favorite bakery with mocha frosting sandwiches, lemon macaroons, and Florentine cookies. I didn't have to share, and I loved being selfish for my special celebration.

In October 2015, I saw Dr. Reid for a checkup, and she said words I thought I'd never hear: "You are excellent and can take the pills as needed." After all of the uncertainty about the long-term outcome of the ablations, Dr. Reid and I thought we'd never get to this healthier place, but we did.

Life's changing for the better. I don't have to spend my days worrying about AFib returning anymore. I don't have to keep waiting for the next bad thing to happen. But the fear's still there, because I've become so used to it. After enduring around thirty cardioversions, I stopped counting procedures, so I can't be sure of the exact number. *I can't believe I've had so many cardioversions and gone to the hospital so frequently. I've canceled so many things. I won't get those friends back.*

The time I took off work illustrates it best: from May 2013 to May 2014, I was out of work for a total of 314 hours (nine weeks) owing to illness and medical appointments. The following June 2014 to May 2015, I was out a total of sixty-three hours (not quite two weeks). From June 2015 to May 2016, I was out of work only a total of nine hours for medical appointments.

I called Mabel to talk after my appointment. "AFib might someday return."

"That's awful," Mabel said. "How are you handling that?"

"Trying not to express my emotions to avoid causing another episode. And I'm really hoping to stop worrying about every flutter I feel. I don't want to check my pulse all the time anymore, either."

"That sucks. I'm sorry that this is how you have to deal with it," she said. "But you must be happy it's over for now?"

"Sure. But I don't know if I'm going on vacation now, until I actually get on the plane. It could come back and then I'd have to cancel."

"That's your life now," Mabel said.

"I appreciate my healthy times more now. But I'm still bitter that not many people have to go through what we do until they're much older. It makes me so mad when old people complain about this stuff since they're just starting to go through it. I know it's new to them, but still."

"I know. This has been our whole lives," she said. "And our families didn't really have any time with us well either."

"We'll never have a time when we're free," I sniffled.

"I know," she said, and we went back to talking about a book we both read.

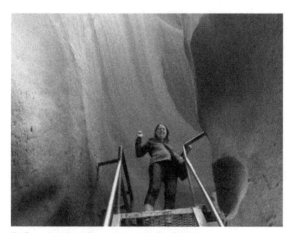

Emily at Antelope Canyon, Age 33 (April 2016)

Strange Happenings

At my December 2015 checkup, Dr. Cole brought up some changes in my recent echo results. "Some of your echo results are better now than when you were a child, but some things are starting to worsen."

Silent, I waited to hear more.

"Your ventricular pump function is excellent, much better than when you were younger. This is because you're taking care of yourself and exercising. Ventricles need to stay in shape like the rest of our muscles."

I nodded, bracing for bad news.

"Compared to your last echo from two years ago, your mitral valve is leaking more now than it was before. Your prior echoes indicated a mild to moderate leak and currently you have a moderate leak. It's a small increase, not too severe, but often as the mitral valve begins to leak, it can progress in a bad direction. We will certainly keep an eye on the leak with your echoes over time. Please don't worry, it's not changing quickly."

I asked, "How concerned should I be that AFib will return and when?"

She responded, "People with some mitral leaking can sometimes have AFib recur later. I don't anticipate anything changing soon. Maybe years down the road, we will probably see a little more mitral leaking, and if it becomes severe, we can talk then about options."

I timidly asked, "Do I need to be concerned?"

She reassured me, "Don't worry! My job is to make sure you are well informed about all the things I assess and am thinking about, but I certainly don't want to alarm you. I don't anticipate any problems anytime soon. Keep exercising. The more active you are, the better. Take on new challenges! You had a great ablation this last time, and things should stay quiet for a long while as long as we keep an eye on the mitral valve."

I went on with my life, feeling reassured that my body was all right, and basically forgot about the conversation for a long time. During 2015–2016, I traveled to New Mexico several times to visit Sam, who was temporarily living there. In April 2016, I emailed Dr. Cole: "Can I go hiking at Antelope Canyon [a slot canyon], in Arizona? The Canyon website advises people with heart conditions to confer with their doctor prior to going because the canyon is rigorous and long, with steep stairs, and is also at a high elevation. I know it might be hard, but I want to try."

Unless there's a firm reason why I can't do something, she usually says yes. She even wants me to do more than I ask.

A few hours later, Dr. Cole replied, "Yes, of course! Have a great time."

I did everything I could to prepare myself and worked intensely with my trainer at the gym to improve on climbing stairs and increase my stamina to make the visit easier. Despite becoming winded at the canyon, I never felt like quitting. On my way up the stairs, I briefly rested because the metal staircase was single file and I couldn't delay others behind me. As I climbed the stairs, I looked to my side to see the orange canyon walls shifting colors in the sunlight, rather than above me to see how much further I had to go. On the top step, I held my arms out and flexed my muscles to flaunt my strength for a triumphant picture, shouting "Hooray!" and pumping my fists.

Of my five planned trips to New Mexico that year, not one was canceled. I had succeeded at a new activity and felt strong. After recovering from AFib, traveling to New Mexico and boxing at the gym, I started to reevaluate past events. *Is it possible for me now to do the things I was restricted from doing all my life? I don't know, but I want to start to find out.*

Softball MVP

In 2016, when I was thirty-four years old, I joined an adult coed softball league. I had never been a part of a team sport, but I always wanted to be, dreaming of the team uniforms, shared experiences, and camaraderie. The same year, more than ten years after Dr. Smith denied my request, I tried indoor rock climbing for the first time. I wasn't great at it, but I was glad I climbed the wall and suffered no ill effects. If I hadn't gone through AFib and learned to treasure my healthy times, I would never have tried rock climbing or softball.

Since I enjoy watching baseball and understand the rules of the game, softball was a good first team sport for me to play. In the summer, I joined a group with games every Saturday against different teams in the same league. On my team, I chose to be the catcher because it felt like a safe position involving less running. Unlike an outfielder, I never ran far to catch a ball. At bat, I could usually hit the ball, but it never went a long distance. I was always tagged out sprinting to first base, so my running ended there. Even though I couldn't contribute much, I tried my best every game because I'm fiercely competitive.

One summer day, it was extremely hot. The team captain was aware of my health conditions.

"I really want to play, Bob, but I'm worried. I don't want to risk AFib returning from exerting myself too much in this miserable heat," I said.

"Should you sit out?"

"I can still catch and hit, but I need a pinch runner."

"Of course. Cait, can you help?"

When I grounded the ball toward the pitcher, he retrieved the ball and tagged out Cait before first base, so I didn't miss out on much. In all the other games, I didn't need any accommodations, and I didn't have to disclose my health history to any of my other teammates.

By the championship game at the end of August, I had made significant progress. Our team was in what was known as the World Series of the league. We had to play two games on the same day to earn the championship title. During the games, I caught a foul ball and tagged a player out—both firsts for me. Twice I was walked to first base when at bat, and from there, I reached home plate after other players successfully batted. I scored three runs. Best of all, I hit a ball all the way to first base—a major accomplishment for me as I usually could hit the ball only halfway back to the pitching mound. Voted the most improved player, I was also voted the All-Star MVP on our championship winning team. I loved being part of a team and giving my best for my teammates. Having people count on me could be nerve-racking, but it also felt good because I was a part of something meaningful.

My teammates and I went out to celebrate after the games, having won gift cards to a local bar. In a once-in-a-lifetime experience when we walked into the bar, all of us wearing our red team T-shirts, everyone cheered for us, giving us high fives, and we strode past them with smiles on our faces singing Queen's "We Are the Champions."

Camp Visit

"Hi, Mabel! Are you up for visiting camp again this year?" I texted.

"Of course! I love going back together to relive our memories and meet the new campers."

"Remember that one camp counselor who wanted to become a heart surgeon?"

"Yes. I wonder what happened to her. I hope she made it."

In August 2016, during my visit to camp with Mabel, a counselor pulled me aside and informed me that they would introduce me to a camper who had undergone a heart and lung transplant. The counselor pointed out that the little girl was doing well and was able to attend camp with only a few restrictions. Her family came to visit and check on her every couple of days (not the norm for others), and she was actively participating in most activities. When I met her, she was hunched over a toy set. Apprehensive and unsure of what to say to her, I reminded myself of what I would want to hear if I were in her position.

"What are you playing? Do you like these toys?" I asked tentatively.

"Yes," she said looking up at me.

"I had heart surgery too, when I was young, and came to this camp." I sat down next to her. "Do you have any questions about anything at all?"

"No, let's play."

I tried to remember what I had asked my older camp counselor all those years ago and realized I hadn't asked her anything about her experience. I merely took in that my counselor was older and thriving, and I hope this little girl I met did as well.

Strange Things Are Happening to Me

The fall of 2016 I still felt strong after my successful summer. When I took a vacation to Europe in October, however, my body began to change. It was a two-week trip, the same length as most of my other worldwide adventures. I chose to climb a glacier at the beginning of my trip to Iceland. After my triumphant summer, thinking that I could handle the challenge with my own precautions in place, I joined a guided tour. *I hope I can do this.* I walked up the steep ice wearing a hard helmet and crampons attached to the bottom of my hiking boots.

One guide, a New Zealander, stayed with me and went at my pace. *I hate inconveniencing people.*

He told me in his exotic accent, "I'm used to guiding the elderly and people with many types of health conditions. Don't worry, we'll make it up the glacier."

As we hiked up, I was behind the group and it was pouring rain. *I didn't know I couldn't keep up with everyone. I wouldn't have booked a group tour otherwise.* Discouraged when I saw people through the sheets of rain so far ahead of me, I thought, *I'll make it eventually. It's so steep and cold. Don't stop me, heart. I'm going to do this!* My guide continued to coach me and kept me moving.

Once I reached the top, I experienced the fun everyone else had. The informational lecture had been missed, but I enjoyed taking pictures of the blue ice, as light blue as the water in the Caribbean, and black volcanic sand. I ran my fingers through the wet sand and collected it in a jar that I brushed my damp hands into. I peeked into crevices in the ice and heard melting water dripping, creating a musical melody like a song. On the way down, the rain had stopped, and I kept up with the group, hearing the information from the missed lecture on glaciers.

When I arrived in London a few days later, I was exhausted. *I don't feel sick. I'm so tired, but nothing else feels wrong. I don't think I can go out. I have to stay in and watch TV. I've never done this on a trip before.* Taking it slow, I stayed in bed and watched television several mornings prior to going out in the afternoon. I napped during the day, much as I did in France in 2014. *My heart's not beating irregularly. I can't get ahead of whatever's happening. Every day, no matter how much I'm resting I wake up feeling run down. I can't bear to eat. Nothing's appealing. I was so looking forward to the grilled tomatoes and now I don't even want a small bite.* Even when I did eat, I never felt energized. *I can't explain any of this. Why do I feel so terrible?* About two weeks after I returned home, I finally felt like myself again with no explanation for what had happened.

Am I not as strong as I hoped I was or thought I was? I never felt that way again, but it was at the back of my mind. That year I also became ill with several colds that lingered for three weeks or more and became much worse before they improved. *This makes no sense! I rarely get colds and if I do, I get better in two weeks. I can't take any cold medicine since they will affect my heart. I'm used to that, but this is miserable. I need help. I can't recover.*

I went to see a doctor about one cold, something I never do. My head was full of congestion and no matter how many times I blew my nose, there was never any relief.

"I figure you can't give me any medicine, but I need help. I need to fly on a plane soon and I don't know how the pressure will affect my ears," I told the doctor.

"There's nothing I can do for you," he said.

This was pointless. Severely coughing on the plane made me feel like I cracked a rib, but my ears were fine.

At every checkup that year with all of my different specialists, I mentioned how I was often becoming sick and having difficulty recovering. None of the doctors could explain it. They didn't investigate further to find any larger concerns.

I had also been gaining weight steadily over the year. My eating habits had not changed, and I was exercising more. No specialist could explain this except to blame it on my age or say it was muscle weight. *I know this isn't right.* A nutritionist tried to help but I merely lost a couple of pounds, nothing compared to what I had gained. *I don't know who else to turn to or what else to do. I'm not having a bad cold year, and it's not age making me gain weight.* I had already seen several specialists and made no progress with a diagnosis or treatment plan. *I don't want to have more tests. If I keep pushing, it's going to be bad news. The doctors are looking out for me; they'd tell me if they found something, and they aren't pushing. If they aren't concerned, I won't be either. My body will tell me if it's getting worse. Then I'll know who to contact for answers.*

AFib's Back

On the morning of Friday, May 12, 2017, at home in Boston, the weekend of Sam's PhD graduation in Washington, DC, I woke up in AFib. *Don't panic, I know what this is. I hope it goes away like it did in April.* After I found my old AFib medication I had long since stopped taking, I took it to try to correct the problem. *Maybe this will help my rhythm go back to normal.* Knowing I couldn't fly for twenty-four hours after having anesthesia if I had a cardioversion and given that I needed to be on a plane the same day, I made the choice not to call Dr. Reid to report my issue. *I can wait to go to the hospital on Monday even if I become tired and run down.* At such a joyous time, I didn't want to worry my family or cause any disturbances.

I followed the schedule for the day with my family, concealing my symptoms. Irregular beating started and stopped. At times, it corrected itself, but then it went back into AFib. The small atrial flutter episodes I experienced in the past had not felt like these larger episodes. As silly as it sounds, my instinct was to hit my chest. Somehow, I hoped that would make the beating stop. It didn't, just as it hadn't helped in the past when I tried the same silly thing.

On Saturday morning, AFib was still there and I was starting to feel worn down and tired. In an email to Dr. Reid, I let her know I'd need an appointment on Monday. I was sharing a hotel room with my parents and they noticed I was taking some medication that wasn't at my routine time. Mom asked quietly, "Is it your eye?"

"No," I said, pausing and rolling my eyes.

It took my parents a moment, but then Mom said, full of worry, "Is it AFib?"

"Yes." I told my parents what had been going on and that I had an appointment scheduled for Monday. I could hear their disappointment as they agreed with my plan. After some more time by ourselves, we left our hotel room and joined Sam to carry on with our graduation plans.

My parents tried to suggest activities with less walking and checked in with me frequently throughout the weekend. Despite becoming more winded on stairs and when walking, I fortunately did not have to miss out on any activities. Mom and Dad told Sam about my AFib, which put a damper on the weekend. My family flew home simultaneously joyous and anxious. I was full of dread because AFib was back. I did not want to return to the EP Lab after such a long absence and go through everything again, but I knew that I would have to face the music on Monday.

On Monday morning, I visited Dr. Reid at the EP Lab, and even though it had been almost two years since my last visit, I was overwhelmed by emotions and memories flooding back. I couldn't help but feel weak and discouraged, as I had felt prior to the second ablation surgery. Dr. Reid and I followed our usual cardioversion routine, and after a single shock, I was back in normal rhythm. We were unsure whether this was a one-time event or if it would recur. Even with the uncertainty, I tried to maintain a positive outlook and focus on the positive aspects of my life.

Big Papi

During this time of my health troubles starting to ramp up again, I had one fantastic experience. I met Red Sox baseball legend David Ortiz, also known as Big Papi. Papi has always been someone I have admired. I say he's like Christmas because he makes everyone happy. He is always in a jovial mood when he is in public, and I used to go to baseball games often just to see him play. Whenever a World Series victory parade snaked through the streets of Boston,

I walked in the crowds alongside him on his winner's float through the length of the city. After my return from Washington, I had the chance to meet him at a signing for his newly published book. I prepared what I wanted to say in advance and wore all of my Big Papi gear to display that I was a true fan.

Not only is Papi an amazing baseball player and person, but his fund, the David Ortiz Children's Fund, provides support for children in the Dominican Republic and in New England who cannot afford critical cardiac services. I feel connected to Papi because he could have chosen any type of charity in the world, but he chose to help children like me. Currently, not many people are aware that children can receive cardiac care at MGH, because they probably think of Boston's Children's Hospital as the go-to place for children. The patients there often have more celebrity visitors and attention in the media. It was especially important for me to acknowledge how much Papi's charity work meant to me when I met him, rather than discussing baseball.

Wearing my fist-size, faux diamond and gold necklace celebrating Papi's 500 Home Runs achievement, handed out at a celebratory game, I got many envious glances as I stood in line at the local bookstore. After zigzagging up a curved staircase and through many rows of books, it was nearly my turn to meet him. My palms were sweating and I had to calm myself. When I got to the front of the line and stood across from Papi, I had a lot I wanted to say in a short period of time. I quickly recited my rehearsed speech. As he signed my book, I said, "I had heart surgery at MGH in 1989 and it's very special what you're doing. There was no one like you when I was there and you're so special!"

He looked up from the book and was taken aback as it was not the usual fan conversation. He replied, "That's very sweet, thank you," and he looked right at me and shook my hand.

My tears flowed freely after I retrieved my signed book and my hands shook as I gloated about my experience to my family.

After much reluctance, I eventually washed my hand later that day and took off my necklace and changed my shirt. *That couldn't have gone any better! It was a dream! It will be a highlight of my life, I'm sure. Even though I was nervous, I was able to tell him how much it means to me that he supports children like me.* When I met Papi, I didn't know I would have heart surgery again in the not-so-distant future.

Life Starts Changing Quickly

A week after Sam's graduation I had a scheduled echo and office visit with Dr. Cole. She knew about the recent AFib episode. She kindly told me, "The echo results exhibit that your heart's not doing well. The leak around your mitral valve ring is becoming worse since your last echo, a year and a half ago. Your heart's more enlarged from the leak around the ring. This affects the electrical heart signals and is probably causing AFib." Dr. Cole kept going, "I think there's a possibility we need to make a change with your mitral valve ring."

What does she mean and what's she going to have me do? I listened to what Dr. Cole said but I didn't dwell on it or truly comprehend the information about ring changes as nothing immediate was needed.

Dr. Cole informed me, "A committee will be formed with your doctors, past and present [many still worked at MGH including my original surgeon], social workers, and nurses who will review your case. We'll all review test results and figure out the best plan of action moving ahead. You can't come to this meeting, but the social workers will advocate for you and try to figure out what would be best in order to improve your condition."

Strangers who don't know me will speak on my behalf? They don't know my values, but I guess they've done this many times before and have my best interests in mind.

"What's the worst-case scenario?" I asked.

"You should be prepared for them to suggest another open-heart procedure."

When I was younger, I was often told if my heart grew much larger than it already was, a new ring might be needed to fit my adult-sized heart to prevent more leaking. This was one of the reasons my surgery was postponed until I was six years old. No one was sure how much I would grow, as cardiac patients don't always thrive and mature to average size, but as it turned out, I am now the tallest woman in my family at 5'6". Mom is 5'4" and Sam is 5'3". I'm very soft-spoken with a childlike voice so sometimes people don't believe I'm tall. When people have only talked with me on the phone, the first thing they say when they meet me in person is, "But you're so big!"

I never thought I'd have to undergo open-heart surgery again. I never became overweight or outgrew my ring. I'm not like the kids at camp or in books who have had multiple surgeries. I'm a one-surgery patient. Other treatments might happen, but I didn't think this would. I'm glad I asked, though. I won't be blindsided or have to make a rushed decision if they do choose this.

"The meeting's scheduled for June 5th, a couple of weeks from now," Dr. Cole said.

That night after speaking to Dr. Cole, I experienced AFib again. I'm sure anticipating the committee's findings was the cause. Luckily, the AFib went away the same night and on a couple of other occasions that week. I continued to go to work and tried not to worry too much because I didn't want AFib to keep recurring, but it was tough to do. Distracted, unable to focus on much, I had difficulty sleeping. I was waiting for the phone call that would seal my fate. Trying to get through my days at work, I hid my anxiety from coworkers by concentrating on independent projects. Staying active, I went on a fundraising walk with Sam for patients with mental health conditions. I didn't feel well, so I managed to walk only one and a half miles of the three-mile course.

On June 5th, I received a voicemail informing me that the meeting had been rescheduled to June 12th owing to Dr. Cole's unexpected out-of-town trip. I endured an extra week of uncertainty and anxiety. In the meantime, I reached out to Dr. Reid to review our treatment plan as I was still experiencing little flutters. Dr. Reid suggested resuming my last AFib medication, propafenone, twice a day to attempt to stop the irregular heartbeats. *I have to have a plan. My trip to Borneo's in October. I planned this a year ago. I won't cancel it. There's nothing else to look forward to. The jungle's scary but I don't want to give up feeling alive when I can.*

On June 12th, one month after Sam's graduation, I worked a partial day and returned home in the afternoon to hear the committee's decision from Dr. Cole. I hurried into the house and sat at my dining room table with paper and pen in hand, ready to take notes. The room was silent except for the ticking of the clock on the wall. Finally, the phone rang, and I answered it right away.

Dr. Cole got right to the point, "The committee reviewed your health history including your mitral stenosis [narrowing of the mitral valve opening that blocks blood flow from the left atrium to the left ventricle], thickening of the leaflets in the valve, and your now significant [upgraded from moderate] mitral leak. The committee has decided you need a new mitral valve. Your mitral ring has a lot of scar tissue around it. The ring needs to be removed because it's not repairable or replaceable. A new mitral valve cannot be implanted through a catheterization procedure. The best course of action is open-heart surgery."

I hurriedly scribbled all my notes about what she was saying. I did not cry or despair because I knew this was a possibility.

"Do I really have to go ahead with this surgery?" I asked. "Instead can I slowly fade away and pass away or stay out of work on long-term disability for the rest of my life?" *Slowly fading away and not working sounds better to me than visible signs of sickness. Being out of work will be great since I hate it there so much.*

Dr. Cole laughed and said gently, "You will gradually deteriorate and work fewer hours, but you will not be ill enough to qualify for long-term disability and you'll have to keep working."

This reminded me of the 2014 trip to France, when I did not enjoy my quality of life because I experienced so much fatigue and little energy to do simple tasks. If I couldn't get out of work, I'd have to keep questioning my options.

"How much chance is there I could feel better after the surgery?"

"There is no percentage I can give to quantify how you might feel later. ... There's another problem to discuss today. We have known we will have to fix your coronary artery when you're in your late thirties or forties."

News to me, as I'd never heard this brought up.

Dr. Cole continued, "By having surgery, we can take care of it while the surgeons are in your heart for the mitral valve. The surgeon on the committee plans to take an artery from your breastbone to improve your blood flow."

This was something I hadn't realized was an issue.

"Dr. Reid also contributed to the meeting. She feels it is unusual for AFib to keep returning. Something else is triggering it after the two ablations, possibly the leaking valve. She thinks a long-term fix is needed. The surgeon can try to revise the ablation lines and touch them up from the inside of the heart. We can't guarantee that AFib won't return from this new procedure, although we can try to eliminate the things irritating your heart from the inside. Dr. Reid feels surgery is best for durability."

Dr. Cole informed me that I could still travel to Borneo in October as planned, as the committee had decided that the surgery was not urgent and could be performed within the next year. Relieved not to have to cancel another trip, I had time to get my affairs in order. The surgery necessitated a three-month absence from work, something I looked forward to. Dr. Cole advised me to set up a follow-up appointment to meet and consult with my new surgeon as a next step.

Once we hung up, I thought about everything she said. *Another surgery isn't so scary. I've lived through one, I can survive another. I trust the doctors, and I'll feel better after it's over. I'm more upset about other things. I don't want bigger scars that I can't hide. It's not an emergency. I can think about my options without rushing. I know I have to have the surgery, but I still have some choices about what's happening to me.*

After reviewing my notes, I called my family on a group conference call to update them. Mom said, "This is not ideal; but if it's what will help you and you'll get better, I'm all for it."

Dad said, "It's what we have to deal with. Trust that the doctors on the committee made the best decision for you. We can ask questions to get to the point where we feel comfortable with the decision to go ahead."

If I wanted to, I could change my decision and not take any action; however, I didn't know of any better options than what the surgeon had proposed. Technology and techniques could advance in the future, but for now this was the best available option.

After the call, I went to my parents' house to be with my family, and I tried to act like everything was fine. We didn't discuss the phone call. Sam, Dad, and I went to the town reservoir to swim. The next day, I took the day off from work to process the news. Negative thoughts crossed my mind, but I pushed them away and avoided dwelling on the unknowns until I had more information. To distract myself, I went on errands with Mom.

The surgeon's office called and arranged a meeting with me, my family, Dr. Cole, and my new surgeon, Dr. Washington. At the meeting, we'd ask all of our questions and learn about what the surgeon had planned.

Preop

Before meeting Dr. Washington, I did an internet search on him. I learned he was new to MGH, although he had many years of professional experience. His name sounded like a soap opera character, which was entertaining. In his online photos he had a genuine smile and tufts of white hair on the sides of his head. I watched videos of him giving talks and felt like I had some idea what he was like ahead of meeting him, which made me less scared. He didn't seem loud or showy, but it was hard to tell what he would be like with patients. I reminded myself not to automatically dislike or distrust him. *He could be kind. He might not treat me like an experiment or medical prize to add to his collection the way others have. He might actually listen to what I have to say and treat me as an individual, not just as another heart he gets to play with.*

On July 5th, my parents, Sam, and I met in the lobby of MGH. We walked past the gift shop and hair salon and took the elevator to a part of the hospital that I had not been to. After walking down a nondescript white hallway, we turned a corner into Dr. Washington's bright and sunny waiting room. I wore my new pair of sea-green sparkly sandals to the meeting to have something positive to look at if I felt overwhelmed. They also helped me to feel like myself and not merely a patient or medical experiment with no choices.

A nurse evaluated me in the exam room, checking my vitals, performing an EKG, and asking me routine questions. Sam accompanied me during the evaluation, and I had the opportunity to ask the nurse my own questions. Afterward, Dr. Washington entered the room, and my defenses instantly went up, as they always do when I meet a new doctor. I smiled and shook his hand, but I refrained from being too chatty to protect myself. Dr. Washington motioned for me to come sit with him at the desk.

Sam left the room, and we walked over to the desk together. Dr. Washington was shorter than me, with a soft warm voice, not intimidating at all. He said we should have a private talk ahead of going into the conference room with my family and Dr. Cole. *Whoa, he actually wants to talk to me.* I lowered my defenses. *He cares about reviewing anything I want to keep confidential. No one ever cares about what I think.* Prior doctors might have been likable and treated me properly, but I never felt I had a choice in what they were doing to me. *Now, I have a voice and a choice.*

I told Dr. Washington the truth. "I don't feel well, but I don't want my family to know." Recounting what happened in Iceland and how I was sick with colds so often over the past year, I brought up that I couldn't recover easily but no one could explain why.

Right away, before he even examined me, Dr. Washington explained, "Your colds and lack of recovery are because your lungs are in a weakened state as a result of your heart health decreasing."

From that moment on, I had confidence in Dr. Washington and completely respected his opinions. I knew something was not right with my body, but my doctors had not dug deeper to discover the reason. My body had been trying to tell me, just like it had with my eye.

After our private discussion, we went into the conference room to meet everyone. As we walked into the room, I sat down at the long table and told the group excitedly, "Dr. Washington can explain my colds." I was happy, and it was a sign my parents could see the appointment was already going well. Normally, I reported on new doctors or my medical appointments in a sad, discouraged voice, but I was acting in the opposite manner this time. I didn't shut down; my comfort with Dr. Washington kept me engaged during the meeting. This ease enabled me to speak up with questions.

Dr. Washington drew diagrams and explained what he proposed to do. "I've never operated on someone with your condition. Very few people around the world have a mitral ring or congenital issues like you, but I have a plan." He kept drawing and detailing his strategy, "There are several goals for your upcoming surgery. Your mitral valve will be removed along with the ring. I will replace it with a new valve."

My mind flashed to echoes where I'd look at the screen to see images of my heart. I could still visualize a tiny beating flap of skin in a dark hole opening and closing my mitral valve, displayed in black and white. Technicians measured blood flow, resulting in bursts of blue, orange, and red flashing across the screen. The ring, which I was told was visible on the screen, would glow, and I pictured it as a plastic wedding ring. The thought of not being able to see it anymore during appointments was unimaginable to me.

I focused back on what Dr. Washington was saying. "You'll also have a maze procedure, a surgical treatment for AFib. I will use different techniques to create scar tissue to stop the pathways causing AFib. Small incisions, freezing, or energy from radio waves, microwaves, are some of the procedures I will use. Additionally, an area where blood clots can form will be destroyed to prevent future risk of stroke. And finally, the anomalous coronary artery, the original problem, originally tied off, will now be bypassed. One of the two arteries that feed tissue around the breastbone will be reconnected to feed the part of the heart that the anomalous artery was meant to feed. For the first time, your heart will hopefully get fed fully. It will restore the original path that was misconnected and then tied off."

At the meeting, we discussed what type of artificial valve I wanted for my mitral valve replacement. Dr. Washington explained the differences between tissue (animal) valves and mechanical valves. "Mechanical valves call for frequent blood tests, daily blood thinner medication, and a modified diet to regulate vitamin K intake. These valves can make noise twenty-four hours a day that might be heard once they are implanted."

I looked at my shoes, thinking *I'll sound like the crocodile in Peter Pan with the constantly ticking clock inside of him. I can't handle that. I'll always know I'm sick, with no relief from the noise, blood tests, or diet modifications.* Both Dr. Cole and Dr. Washington agreed that a mechanical valve might not be the best option for me, considering my aversion to blood tests and desire to minimize medical intrusions into my life. Although this surgery to implant a mechanical valve could be the only open-heart surgery I'd ever need for the rest of my life, in the unlikely case that it failed and needed to be serviced or replaced, it would necessitate another open-heart surgery, which carries more risks than a tissue valve replacement or correction. On the other hand, a tissue valve has a lifespan of ten to twelve years and needs to be replaced when it becomes worn down, depending on the case. It can be replaced a total of three times during a person's lifetime. Unlike a mechanical valve, a new tissue valve replacement can sometimes be inserted into the heart through the groin, eliminating the need for open-heart surgery. There would be no promise of that method being an option. It wouldn't be an option the first time it was implanted, so I carefully weighed all of these factors before deciding. As an animal lover, the thought of having an animal valve implanted also troubled me.

Dr. Washington said in his easy-going manner, "You can change your mind on the type of valve you want until a few days before the surgery."

Phew. This is a lot. I have to decide between having more open-heart surgeries resulting in thicker chest scars versus a reduced quality of life. This is a big decision I have to make on my own.

After my questioning, Dr. Washington said, "There will be no new life restrictions placed on you, except for what the mechanical valve dictates, and no new annual tests to monitor either type of valve. You still have to have echoes and EKGs but nothing you're unfamiliar with."

I nodded and he continued, "You should feel better than you ever have after the surgery as a result of the improvements I plan to make."

I didn't think much about this remark, assuming that Dr. Washington meant that I would feel better without the constant effects and worries of AFib. Wanting simple outcomes, I never had high expectations. My hope was that the surgery would help me lose weight and stop the colds. I didn't want to dwell on the details of the procedure or the associated risks because they weren't my primary concerns. My main focus was on deciding which valve to choose.

"What about my trip to Borneo?" I asked, as my parents rolled their eyes, prioritizing my health. Because I was an adult Dr. Washington and Dr. Cole could not tell me outright not to go to Borneo, but they thought it was unwise.

"There are no immediate risks to waiting to do the surgery since there's nothing we can predict might suddenly go wrong."

The terrain would be rough and hilly, and the weather would be hot and extremely humid. *I'm not admitting how hard this will be.* "I still want to go. I researched several medical facilities already. What should I do if something unexpected happens? What if I have AFib again? What if my heart failure worsens?" Until the meeting with Dr. Washington, I didn't even know I was in moderate heart failure, which was a surprise to me.

Dr. Washington said, "We'll give you a list of colleagues to call if something happens in case of an emergency or if you feel terrible."

Now I feel as prepared as I can for every possible scenario. After the consultation, my family and I returned to our respective homes, trying to process all of the information we had been given. The next day, I called other hospitals to inquire about obtaining second opinions regarding my treatment options. While I wasn't particularly interested in doing so, Sam urged me to seek additional opinions from other surgeons to ensure that I made the best decision possible given my rare condition. My case was so uncommon, it wasn't like I could look specifics up in books or online. The other hospitals' responses were overwhelming and involved numerous tests to determine the best course of action. Instead of going to another hospital and undergoing additional tests, I decided to ask Dr. Washington to consult with his colleagues to obtain their opinions.

Dr. Washington sought the opinions of cardiologists at the Mayo Clinic and Cleveland Clinic, both of whom agreed with his plan to replace my mitral valve, perform a bypass, and carry out the modified maze procedure. I then asked Dr. Washington to consult with my first surgeon, Dr. Hunter, from 1989, who was still working at MGH. Dr. Hunter emailed me and said, "Dr. Washington's plan is perfect. He has devoted a huge part of his career to dealing with problems like yours. What he is suggesting is really the contemporary way to deal with your situation, and I agree with him." Dr. Hunter's endorsement assured me more than anything else could have. He was the only doctor I could still contact who had seen inside my heart in reality, rather than on an ultrasound screen, and I felt confident after communicating with him. Dr. Smith also confirmed that it was best to address my mitral valve issue as soon as possible.

Making My Decision

I've never had anything taken out of my body during surgeries, only things put in to help it function better. I don't feel so good about giving away a part of my body that I can't ever get back. My valve and ring have been a part of me so long, it will be hard to let them go. They make me unique. I can't imagine what life would be like without them. I better ask Dr. Washington my questions to understand this better.

Dr. Washington always responded quickly to my emails full of questions and concerns, and even called me one Sunday to talk. He never rushed me and he thoroughly answered everything, no matter how trivial it might have seemed to him. I tried to bargain with Dr. Washington about getting a new valve, suggesting the implantation of a 3D printed valve, but he informed me that it was not an option at the time. While 3D valves are starting to be used in France, I would have to wait for the technology to become more reliable before considering it.

Accepting a new valve as my way forward, I seriously began my decision-making process to choose which type to get. I didn't want to rush my decision, but I also wanted to make it quickly so I wouldn't have to dwell on it and could move on. Researching on the internet for other people's stories and experiences with the two different types of valves was informative. I also consulted with my doctors. Dr. Reid said, "Being on blood thinners this young isn't a good idea. Getting a tissue valve and waiting for future technology is better."

I decided on the tissue valve, as my quality of life would, I hoped, be better than with the restrictions a mechanical valve would place on me. The surgery was scheduled for November 6th, a week after my return from Borneo. I figured I would need time to recover from the trip, return to work to tie up loose ends, and get my life in order prior to my incapacitation.

I sent out an email on July 11th, to inform my family and friends about the news:

> I have some updates about my health. This summer I found out that I need to have open-heart surgery again. Last time I did this I was six, so it's been almost thirty years! I'm lucky that I didn't need it sooner.
>
> I am not in any pain or doing poorly or having any emergency (it was my decision when to do this surgery). It's just that some things from when I was young need updating to help me to feel better and keep from getting worse or making me feel bad. I am still at work full-time and will be until surgery. ...
>
> I am not scared, worried or concerned. I will be at MGH with many of the same doctors I've had my entire life. Please try to not worry either.
>
> I can still go to Borneo in September so picture me there if you get worried.

Mom created an email group of close family and friends to update them on my health. She sent them updates on all the steps of my medical journey and informed them about my upcoming procedure.

Many people responded back to both Mom and me. Some emails were more reassuring than others. It surprised me how others perceived me during this time because I didn't feel the way they thought I did. People called me brave, strong, courageous, a trooper, and a fighter. Many were unaware of how much I had actually gone through in recent years and how I truly felt about the upcoming surgery. From the emails, I realized how people who had not experienced chronic illness viewed my situation.

My family friends who live in France, the Gees, who have known me since I was a baby and are my trusted friends, wrote, "I am amazed by the cool way you are able to manage while sailing through basic decisions."

Relatives wrote to me, "Sorry you have to undergo this, but I guess after thirty years the warranty must be running out." Other relatives wrote, "We're very sorry that you are approaching another operation. You have a wonderful attitude regarding this development, and we admire you for it."

Mom's friends wrote to her, "Although I cannot imagine your stress level, it certainly sounds like now is the time."

A relative wrote, "Hang in there, brave Emily. I hope all goes well and you are feeling good and strong again soon."

It was hard reading all of the emails even though they were supportive and understanding because they couldn't truly know what I faced. Sometimes I wanted to shout that I didn't feel brave or strong. It might have been nice to read an email like, "This is terrible!" Saying they were sorry and wishing for the best felt like glossing over the situation.

I realized that people were telling me that I was brave to ease their own feelings. If they felt I could get through this experience, then they wouldn't have to worry about me as much. They could go on as if this was a normal occurrence in my life. I valued their emails a great deal, but I never shared how I honestly felt, as it would have been too much for them. I craved a different type of support, and I found myself inept at explaining how it actually felt to have to go through yet another surgery. Even with my closest family and friends, like my parents and Mabel, I couldn't communicate my feelings effectively.

It is not a matter of choice for someone who has been sick most of their life to be strong. Being strong is a necessity for survival. Is it brave to do something you have to do? I didn't think so. Should I give up and wither away instead? My conditions are not fatal. I could give up and stop fighting, but I would continue to suffer. I could tell myself I was brave and strong for doing this, but the truth is, it was not really my choice. I had to do it—and it sucked. I have no choice but to find a way through my predicaments in order to feel better and improve my quality of life. Healthy people may see this as a choice, but for me, it is a requirement. Surgeries may be grueling, but not doing anything to treat my problems would be problematic forever.

Coming to Terms with What Is Ahead

Dad and I had a serious phone conversation one night after we informed our family and friends. He said, "We'll get through this surgery like we have the other ones."

"I feel like people are treating me like I am the walking dead once they find out about this," I said sadly. "Lots of photographs are being taken because people fear I won't be around much longer."

Dad reassured me, "We all might act funny during this hard time, but no one doubts you will be fine in the end." This advice helped to keep me calm.

Whenever I spoke about what was going on, I stayed outwardly positive. I cried only a few times alone. Inside, I was not freaking out because I had time before doing anything. The surgery was months away, and I always feel better when I can prepare and not rush into momentous events. When my mind wandered, thinking about frightening things like pain or scars, I tried to stop thinking about them by keeping busy. I tried not to obsess over the medical details or worry myself by reading anything online. I didn't dwell on understanding every little thing the surgeon would do or all of the medical information given to me.

I also tried to focus on the positives, like going to Borneo, but I couldn't always do it. At night, strange, sharp, and sudden pain would shoot through my teeth. I was clenching my jaw and grinding my teeth because the subconscious stress was manifesting physically. After my dentist reviewed the issue and told me it was all in my mind, I stopped grinding my teeth, and the pain went away. I didn't get much sleep as I stayed up late into the evening to prepare for my absence around the house and trip to Borneo. To avoid dwelling on the same things, I functioned on autopilot by making an out-of-office guide for my work colleagues, creating a to-do list ahead of surgery for me, and listing all of the concerns I wanted to review with Dr. Washington.

Waiting for the surgery to take place, I ate foods I had not allowed myself because they were fattening. I treated myself to a feast at Olive Garden and ate numerous breadsticks, salad, lasagna, and ravioli, a treat I hadn't indulged in since college. I also used my special soaps and lotions purchased throughout the years on vacations and at special events that I had been saving. Although it was unlikely that the surgery would turn out badly, I didn't want to regret the things I hadn't done, eaten, or used in my life.

AFib Returns, Yet Again

Because of the stress, I experienced more frequent AFib episodes. I had high beats and then they sometimes dissipated on their own. Often these irregular beats were atrial flutter that I had experienced previously. One afternoon I went sailing with Dad while I had AFib. We went on the Charles River with his college alumni group on a sunny day, and saw the tall buildings gleaming and reflecting in the deep blue water as we sailed around the city. *Don't get up to walk, or take a turn steering. It might make the AFib worse.* I pretended to tan on the bench (instead of obviously staying still to rest) so Dad wouldn't become worried. *Another fun memory will always be associated with AFib. This reminds me of all the places I've had AFib here and on vacation. I don't want to be experiencing such an unpredictable life again.*

I went in to see Dr. Reid on Monday, July 17th, for a cardioversion. We went through our usual routine, but when I woke up, I could still feel my heart pounding. *It didn't work! This has never happened. I'm scared.*

Everything was the same for this episode. Why didn't it work? I stared at the monitor, seeing my pulse was still extremely high as Dr. Reid arrived at my bedside. *I'm in for some bad news. She rarely comes by after cardioversions. Something serious is going on.*

Dr. Reid told me tenderly, "The cardiologists tried a few times to shock your heart. Your heart decided to be stubborn and had other ideas. It won't convert so we can see how the week goes and if you can cardiovert on your own."

I nodded, still unsure why this was happening, but there were no answers. Dr. Reid put me back on my AFib medications.

"If there's no change to the heart rhythm, come back on Friday to try the procedure again."

I agreed to this plan, depressed that I had relapsed back to life on the medications I had so happily been free of for so long.

During the week, I emailed Dr. Reid suggesting another ablation so I could go to Borneo in October and have the surgery in November. I could feel my trip slipping away. She replied, "We can't do another ablation. We will have to wait for the surgery and continue to try the cardioversions when possible."

On Friday, July 21st, I went to work for a half day and went to the hospital in the afternoon. In advance of entering the EP Lab I met my parents in the hall instead of inside the lab. Before I had even walked into the hospital, I felt defeated. I'd never felt a sense of dread or not wanting to go into the lab or hospital. Confident I could be helped, I had always gone in with a positive attitude. *I can't bear going into the lab.* I told my parents I wanted to go to the restroom in another part of the building. *I don't want to go through any more cardioversions that don't work. I have to get myself together.*

As soon as I entered the restroom, I burst into tears. No one was at the sink, but I rushed into a stall to have some privacy. *Stay calm.* I took some deep breaths. *You have to come out of here and be on time for your appointment.* I stayed there for a couple of minutes, not wanting my parents or anyone else to see me being so emotional. After drying my tears, I left the stall. When I rejoined my parents in the hall, I struggled to keep myself from crying. Although my parents were sympathetic, we had to enter the lab to find out what was going on.

My heart had been beating irregularly on and off, and I had a feeling I wouldn't qualify for a cardioversion. When the nurse called me back from the waiting room to the procedure room, and I left my parents, I began to cry again. I didn't want to go through the usual routine without knowing what the EKG indicated first. Before going into the bathroom to change, I told the nurse I wanted to talk to Dr. Reid. I stood outside the bathroom, and when Dr. Reid saw me, she noticed how unusual I was acting and took me to her office, full of concern. We spoke privately away from the lab and the commotion inside.

"I think I'm in atrial flutter. I don't want to do all of this for nothing," I cried.

Dr. Reid completely understood my hesitation. An EKG in her office revealed normal rhythm. We couldn't do a cardioversion. Dr. Reid said, "In the future, we can always try the procedure again if the beats start up again and stay that way for a longer time; however, you need to think about how you are feeling emotionally and physically in general. Please consider your options about the surgery and Borneo." If what she had said had come from any other doctor I might not have listened, but I trusted her and knew she would never pressure me one way or another about a decision on how to move forward. We both thought being in normal rhythm was temporary.

My parents drove me back to work that afternoon because I did not want to be alone at home with my thoughts. I sat at my desk, running reports, keeping myself distracted. After a week of abnormal rhythm, I felt physically and mentally exhausted. Throughout the day and night, my heart continued to beat irregularly. The pounding kept me awake, like old times, and I got very little sleep. Early the next morning, lying in the dark in my bed, with my chest thudding and pounding in my ears, I made the decision to have my surgery earlier and to cancel my trip to Borneo.

I called my parents to let them know. After the call, I emailed Dr. Washington to request a new surgery date in early August. He promptly called me and agreed with my decision. "Call or email me anytime. My office will follow up on Monday with a scheduled surgery date." Rather than feeling nervous in anticipation, I was relieved. Everyone was so accommodating it made the change in plans go very smoothly.

On Monday morning, I went back to work. Walking from the bus stop to the office was more challenging than ever, with my heart thumping and I felt the need to rest after short distances. I knew I couldn't keep commuting every day until the surgery. I talked to my manager, and we decided that day would be my last day in the office before my medical leave. I could work remotely for a few days at home to finish my projects and tasks. Since I had already been preparing to be out in November, all that was left for me to do was organize a few more files ahead of my departure. I spent the rest of the day training colleagues for my absence and waiting for the call from Dr. Washington's office with the new surgery date.

The Final Few Weeks

My surgery was scheduled for August 9, 2017, and everything proceeded quickly. This was twelve weeks after the AFib episode in May, which occurred during Sam's graduation. Instead of dwelling on my feelings, I focused on what was right in front of me, working from home. Two weekends ahead of the surgery, my family and I went to Vermont to celebrate Sam's thirtieth birthday and my thirty-fifth, which we had previously planned. The atmosphere was somber, and although no one explicitly mentioned the possibility of a bad outcome, or did anything like crying in front of me, the worries were palpable. The trip became a kind of death-cation. My picture was being taken much more frequently and I won arguments often.

"I want to have pasta," I said to my family during the nightly dinner choice debate.

"Sure," Sam agreed.

That's strange. She always wants something fancy. Why's she letting me win … oh. That's also why we sat in the park instead of going on the walk she wanted.

Dr. Washington advised us that the risks of the upcoming surgery included a one percent risk of stroke and one percent risk of death. I didn't like to think about the risks. Although my family was anxious, we tried to stay positive so that we could have a good time, not knowing if it would be the last birthday I celebrated or our last family vacation together.

Even though I wasn't feeling my best, I had a fun birthday celebration and was glad to be away from home. I indulged in lots of sweets, and we drove over the Canadian border for an Italian birthday dinner. Although I usually enjoy canoeing, I didn't feel up to it on this trip and instead watched Sam and Dad canoe without me from a chair on the beach. Since I was feeling more tired than usual, I didn't walk as much and went to bed early. Discouraged, I couldn't push myself and wanted to be in the best shape possible for the surgery.

Two nights in a row in Vermont, we all crammed into the car, driving around at dusk to look for a moose. My family and I were hoping to spot a moose as they are known to frequent the area we were staying in. Prior to the trip, I had never had much interest in moose, but everyone was hopeful to see one on this vacation. We drove through the streets, stopping to wait in wooded areas, but we didn't see a moose the first night. The second night, on my birthday, we went out again to look for one. *If we see a moose, I'll survive the surgery.* Eventually, after driving around and patiently waiting, we saw one. The brown giant lumbered down the street in front of the car and we saw its mammoth form disappear between thick trees after a few seconds. *Everything's gonna work out.* I can't explain how I had such confidence. It wasn't faith in a higher power; it was more faith in myself and my medical team. *If I were going to die, I'd be dead by now. I'm ready for the surgery.*

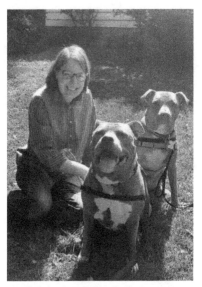

Blueberry and Maxi, with Emily, Age 35
(September 1, 2017)

The Second Surgery

"Please remember how important it is to me to minimize my scar," I said to Dr. Washington at our preop appointment. *Mabel said scars are a roadmap showing all the brave things you've been through, but I don't feel that way. They're a red flag, directing attention to my health problems.*

Looking at the floor, remembering, I said, "I went to a Red Sox game once a few years ago and a guy flirted with me and asked me out. When I said no, he said, 'You know, I noticed your scar so I know something's going on with you.' It was humiliating." I sighed thinking back on this memory and looked back at Dr. Washington. "And on TV, characters who have heart surgery often retain their scars only in the initial episode and they're never seen again. There's no normalization for audiences. So my scar's my biggest concern."

Dr. Washington replied, "I completely understand, and I will try my best to make it as minimal as possible."

During our meeting, I recounted events I remembered from my first surgery at age six that I didn't want repeated. I said emphatically, "No daily blood tests in my arm every morning. I can't go through the experience again, and chest tube removal day has to go smoothly." Clear on my musts and must nots, we came to compromises and agreements the best we could. "It's crucial I still take my eye drops even if I'm not alert to my surroundings during recovery. I know everyone will be focused on my heart, but we have to care for my eye, too."

Dr. Washington took notes to ease my apprehension.

"I don't think I'll need these things, but here are my signed Living Will and Healthcare Proxy documents," I said as I handed the required documents over. At my prompting, we discussed end-of-life options if I needed to be placed on life support and documented my choices.

"You can change your mind about which type of tissue valve you want until a couple of hours before the procedure," he said. Then Dr. Washington told me how my surgery and recovery should go if all went according to plan. He said, "I'll call you the night prior to the procedure so we can discuss any last-minute concerns."

After our meeting, I apprehensively went to have tests performed in the hospital. I needed an MRI so Dr. Washington could have an up-to-date model of my heart and circulatory system. With the model, he could plot out the procedures he planned to do. I went into the dressing room to change into a hospital gown for the MRI. As I stood in front of the mirror looking at myself, I realized *this is a good opportunity to take a photo of my body*. I took a full-length picture of my chest and stomach scars in the mirror. *Don't forget how they look. You might not ever look the same again.* Trying to burn the image into my brain, I left the dressing room. After the MRI, X-rays, and blood tests, I was free to return home after a full day spent at the hospital.

The Final Countdown

On Sunday night, I went to my last scheduled event, a Roaring Twenties party at the Crane Estate in Ipswich, Massachusetts. The vast Tudor Revival mansion, with a view of the ocean and acres of lush green grass, was the perfect venue for the event. I wore a beaded black period dress, with a silver headband and black feather in my hair, and enjoyed the distraction of looking at the costumes and cars. The one negative of the night was that my legs became covered in bug bites that frequently itched. Interestingly, after the surgery, they no longer itched, as my body had more important parts to heal.

The last days before the surgery, I focused on completing tasks that I could do at that moment and tried to ignore the future. I caught up on TV shows and took care of chores around the house, such as vacuuming and changing the sheets on my bed, which I might not be able to perform later.

Superstitious, I had the need to control what I could. I told my family that I wanted to experience my surgery as closely as possible to how I had experienced it before. Since my first surgery was a success, I thought the second would be, too, if I repeated the same routine. We went over my memories, and my family agreed to do everything they could to repeat my experiences. One of the experiences we could not repeat was the admission day. It was not necessary to check into the hospital prior to the surgery as I had done in the past. Instead, I would check in on the morning of the procedure. To make everything easier, my family decided it would be best for all of us to stay together in a hotel next to MGH.

On Wednesday, August 8th, at my condo, I completed packing for my recovery period at my parents' house. After taking my time to ensure everything was in order, I drove to their house after lunch. While at their house, I kept myself occupied by watching TV and attending to unanswered emails. At 3 p.m., it was time to head to the hotel in Boston. From the back seat of the car, I replayed sitting in the front seat in my mind so it would be similar to the first time I had made this same drive for surgery.

We took the subway into town and checked into our hotel. Our room was on a high floor facing the hospital with Fenway Park in the distance. The pungent smell of the recently cleaned carpet filled the room, as did the sound of the loud air conditioning window unit. I sat on the bed on the crisp white sheets, looking out the window while waiting for Sam, who arrived shortly after check-in, and then it was time for dinner. I elected to walk to dinner instead of taking the subway because I didn't know how long it would be until I could walk long distances again. We went to the North End for an Italian meal and spent some time browsing menus until we finally settled on a restaurant. Delicious tempting aromas of garlic and marinara sauce filled the air, but I wasn't hungry and opted for a Caesar salad and a few bites of pasta. As I watched my family eat, my phone rang. Dr. Washington called, as promised, to go over any last-minute concerns.

To have some privacy and quiet, I stepped outside of the restaurant to speak with him. As we spoke, my teeth chattered with nerves, but I tried to speak normally.

"You can report to the hospital at 9 a.m. No food after midnight tonight," he said.

I returned to the restaurant after our conversation and relayed the information to my family. I had a few more bites of my last meal before surgery.

That night, I shared a bed with Sam, and we spoke quietly as our parents slept. We reviewed a couple of concerns I had and talked about the future before Sam fell asleep after staying up pretty late with me. As I lay on my side, I watched the lights of Fenway Park shining during and after that night's baseball game from the window next to my bed. The lights continued to shine until they were shut off around 2 a.m. I tried to sleep but kept waking up. Whenever I couldn't sleep, I reviewed in my mind all that I wanted to be sure to tell the nurse taking care of me the following day.

Surgery Time

Wednesday, August 9, 2017, was surgery day. When I woke up in the morning, I lay in bed with my eyes closed, listening to my family getting ready. The comforting sounds of Dad brushing his teeth, Sam brushing her hair, and Mom packing her purse made it feel like an ordinary day, but I knew it wasn't. I could smell their leftover food and bitter coffee, but it didn't make me hungry or upset that

I couldn't eat. After a few minutes of lying in bed pretending I was asleep to have some last moments of normalcy, I got up to take my preop shower. Everyone said good morning as I passed by them in the room, but no one was particularly cheery or chatty. The hospital had provided me with disinfectant soap I needed to bathe with the morning of the procedure. As I scrubbed myself, I said goodbye to the body I knew so well, trying to imprint its image in my mind. Looking one last time at my scar after I stepped out of the shower. I got dressed for the day in clothes I didn't care about and removed my jewelry. It was my final time alone before everything commenced. Anxious only about the IV and needing to remember what I wanted to say to the nurses, I felt resigned and ready to go.

My family and I left the hotel and started to walk to the hospital. Everyone was sullen and making small talk. Sam had not yet eaten breakfast and she let me choose her a decadent pastry at a bakery to eat after I was in surgery. It was a good distraction on the walk over. As we approached the last sidewalk before the hospital entrance, I decided to run. I wasn't sure if I would be able to run again if things went badly. *I might not be as able-bodied again as I am right now. Or, if I do feel different later, I want to remember what it feels like to run in the body I've always known.*

I ran a little way down the sidewalk as fast as I could with Sam running behind me. *I can pass her, if I push myself. I haven't done that in a long time and I'm only out of breath, no AFib.*

My parents walked briskly to catch up. We turned the corner and approached the familiar driveway leading to the hospital's revolving doors. I didn't feel like crying because I knew I was going in for help to fix a problem, rather than fighting a disease with unknowable outcomes. *Be strong for everyone.* We entered the hospital lobby together and took the elevator to the admissions area, which was no longer where it had been thirty years ago. Instead, it was a vast room with a check-in desk and multicolored seats everywhere, more like a hotel lobby. All the patients who needed surgery that day at MGH were present with their companions. There was no sectioning of the room by procedure or patient age, so it was impossible to tell why everyone was there.

The receptionist put a hospital bracelet on me and informed me that there would be a short wait. While I waited, I texted with Mabel and, after saying goodbye to her, I tried to stay distracted by looking out the window and talking with my family. The room was quiet and tense, with the sound of talk-show hosts blaring on the televisions.

Eventually, someone called my name to take me to the procedure and I requested my family come with me. The nurse explained that they could join me later in the preop area, but I went in alone first to get ready.

I was taken to a spacious hospital floor with open bays and curtains for privacy, similar to those in an ER, with a nurse's station in the center. My bay was at the end of the hall, in the corner, and noticeably larger than the others. I wasn't sure if it was by chance, because of my age, or because of the procedure I was about to have, but I appreciated the VIP treatment. Being in a quiet and isolated area, I wasn't disturbed by any distressing events occurring in nearby bays. As I was being prepped, I had several large, open windows to gaze out of. After I answered some questions, I changed into a gown.

My family came into the room as the anesthesiologist asked, "Do you want to take some medication to stay calm?"

"No," I said, because I did not notice myself feeling anxious. I felt mostly fine.

The doctor raised his eyebrows in surprise and tried to convince me otherwise. It was the first time I cried that day and I repeated I didn't want it. I cried not because of the pressure from the doctor to do something I didn't want to do; rather it was a feeling of losing control. *I don't know what the medicine will make me feel like or do. I have to be aware of all decisions going on around me.* Sam and Mom thought I should take the medicine and their insisting made me more emotional.

The anesthesia the doctor would administer to put me to sleep had some relaxing drugs in it, so I said between sniffles, "I'd rather wait. If you think that I'm starting to act anxious you can tell me and I'll take the drugs." Once we settled that I didn't have to take any medication until later, I stopped crying.

Events moved quickly after that. The nurse informed me that it was time to be taken downstairs to the operating room to have my IV inserted. My family had to leave; they gave me hugs and said their goodbyes. Sad at first, I almost instantly stopped crying as I knew I would see them again in what would feel like no time at all after I woke up from the surgery.

Sitting up in the bed, I was wheeled to the surgical floor of the hospital. Being rolled on a gurney down the hallway for any procedure feels like taxiing on a plane runway. There's no way to predict how long the nerve-racking journey will take. It's like looking out of the small window to see the long runways stretching before you or peering through the metal railing slots on your gurney to see the white hallways surrounding you. There is no control or knowing what will happen; only the final destination is certain.

I arrived on the surgical floor, where there were paintings of the ocean and sea creatures on the swinging doors leading into the OR. My bed was placed directly across from the doors. As I waited for the next steps and sat alone looking around, I had some time to think. *I don't expect to get much out of this. I can't imagine feeling better than I have in the past. I won't be able to do anything new, I'm sure.* I had no concept of what feeling better would be like. In 2002, I had written a paper for a class in college and said, "In the future my health will not change enough for me to participate in any activity I have always dreamed of." I don't remember what I meant at the time, maybe a trip to a challenging destination at high elevation or playing a sport with friends. On surgery morning, I thought, *I don't want to feel crummy again like when I experienced AFib so frequently. I hope for a discreet scar and less unpredictable illness in the future.*

Shortly after my time alone, a surgical nurse inserted my IV with the help of an ultrasound machine to find my vein. A kind nurse dressed in dark navy scrubs approached me and explained the procedure, along with what was planned once they opened me up. Dr. Washington came by to see me, and I barely recognized him. Instead of wearing a simple surgeon's cap on his head, he had on a hood that covered his head and the sides of his face and neck, leaving only the front of his face visible. Although our visit was brief, it was reassuring to see him and we reconfirmed, for one last time, which type of valve he would implant. He went to tell my family they would begin shortly and he told Sam, "I hope I can not only do the job but also put a smile on your face."

The surgical nurse took me into the cold OR, where trays of metal instruments and tools were lined up around the room. Several doctors were gathered in a corner, but they didn't acknowledge my arrival. The nurse placed an oxygen breathing mask on me and told me it was time to go to sleep. The familiar smell of oxygen, sweet and sticky like raisins, filled my nostrils. I remained calm and felt no pain when the anesthesia was administered, thanks to the numbing injection in my vein. I didn't fall asleep right away. While I waited and looked around, sadly, there were no doctors or nurses watching me fall asleep, talking to me, or smiling at me as Dr. Reid had for all of my most recent procedures. I didn't like being alone, but the next time I woke up it would all be over. I lay my head down as the dizziness started and I went to sleep.

While I Was Sleeping …

When the procedure began or how long it took is a mystery to me, but I know my family spotted Dr. Washington in the cafeteria when they went to have lunch. Based on that, I would say that the surgery probably commenced around noon or 1 p.m. and was over by evening. The duration of open-heart surgery is determined by how long patients can be on the heart/lung machine; the surgeon has to work within that time frame, and the shorter the better.

The hospital staff gave my family many status updates throughout the day. In the early evening, they transferred me to the Cardiac Surgical Intensive Care Unit (CSICU). Around 7 p.m., Dr. Washington updated my family on everything he had done during the surgery. During the procedure, he performed the maze ablation to, he hoped, eliminate my AFib, and he destroyed an area of my heart where clots could form to reduce the risk of blood clots and stroke. While attempting to undo the artery that had been tied off for bypass, he discovered that it was unnecessary. He tested my blood supply and found that it was sufficient, so he concluded that no changes were necessary.

Dr. Washington removed my mitral ring and replaced my valve with a tissue valve using the largest size available, which could allow for future replacement procedures through the catheterization technique. Most important, Dr. Washington delivered the astonishing news to my family that, for the first time since the heart attack I had as an infant, my mitral valve did not leak. It was an amazing achievement, and my family had no idea what it would mean for my quality of life going forward, but it could only suggest a promising future.

After the surgery, Dr. Washington continued to keep my family updated on my progress, but I was not yet out of the woods. My cognitive functions would need to be tested when I woke up about six hours later in the evening. After quickly eating dinner, my family returned to the CSICU waiting room, where they met Tom, my CSICU nurse for the night. Later, when they saw me, they described me as having looked pale but okay. They could tell I was not breathing naturally, but rather was relying on machines. I remained stable, and my family eventually went back to the hotel to get some rest.

Until the early morning, Sam called Tom in the CSICU every hour to check on my condition and to see if I had woken up. She wanted to keep her promise of being there when I regained consciousness. Tom informed her that I had responded well to a basic orientation test, indicating positive signs for my cognitive functioning. It would take some time, however, for the breathing tube to be removed, and I wouldn't be able to receive visitors until the next morning.

Waking Up in a Changed Body

On the morning of August 10th, I woke up in the CSICU. My lower body reclined, and my chest and head were propped up on pillows like I was relaxing on a couch. As I took in my surroundings, I noticed that the room was exceedingly bright. It was around 4 or 5 a.m., although I wasn't sure of the exact time. Immediately, I gagged on the tube in my throat helping me breathe. Tom sat at a desk nearby and hadn't heard me wake up. I didn't register any pain or much discomfort aside from the gagging. *Pay attention to me and help me!* My arms were tied to the bed rails, and I banged the cuffs on the side of the bed to get his attention. He rushed over and injected me with antinausea drugs and I fell back to sleep.

Every five to ten minutes, I woke up gagging and glanced at the black hands of the clock, feeling infuriated that more time had not passed. Tom continued to administer drugs to alleviate my discomfort, and I would fall back to sleep. After a while, it was time for the removal of my breathing tube. He explained the process and made sure I could comprehend his instructions. Glad to have the tube removed, I didn't mind the coughing the procedure caused or having to use my limited energy to expel it. Tom asked me questions to assess if I had any brain damage. He asked me where I was, and I responded, "In hell." *I know this is wrong, but I hope he laughs.* He did and I quickly told him where I actually was and readily answered the rest of his questions.

Tom let me know my family had been calling and checking up on me and would be coming into the room soon. *My chest feels heavy and numb. I can't feel my hospital gown or blankets on it.* Just like in childhood, I gulped water off small sponges and drank too much and choked.

"There's some people that would like to see you," Tom said as my family came into the room single file. They stood by my bedside, smiling at me and inquiring about how I was feeling during a brief visit that I do not recall in much detail. Mom brought my eye drops, which I took with Tom's assistance. I was relieved that I was aware enough to remember to do it and was taking care of myself. Sam noticed I was suffering and needed more pain medication, but there was a delay in receiving it. She sternly spoke to the nurses and it was administered.

Time went by and I was wheeled in the bed up to my room on the hospital floor. I was checked into the Cardiac Surgery Step Down Unit. Lifted up out of the bed in the same contraption that had been used for ablations, I was placed into my new bed. It was expected I would stay about a week on this floor to recover and then go home if all went well.

My two-person room was situated at the end of the hallway, away from the noise emanating from the nurses' desk. My room-mate was behind a curtain, so I never saw her. She didn't make much noise, although she received a constant stream of visitors who walked by my bed to get to hers.

My bed was the closest to the door, so I could see, to my right, all the comings and goings outside in the hall, as the doctor's lounge was across the way. On the opposite side of my bed, a whiteboard hung on the wall displaying information such as the date, scheduled appointments, and nurses' details. My family came into the room after a little while.

As the day wore on, my new nurse, Lynn, provided me with information on the various postsurgical restrictions I was to follow.

Among them, I learned that I could not lift my arms above my head, and it was mandatory for me to maintain an upright chest posture at all times. This was because my sternum had been broken during the surgery to gain access to my heart, and it would take four to six weeks to fully heal. Feeling like my chest was caving in and crushing me when I lay flat or was in a reclined position, I was required to sit at a vertical angle to sleep.

Lynn also introduced me to cough pillows. She let me know, "As the anesthesia wears off you might start coughing as your body tries to expel all of the gunk inside your lungs. The pain will be excruciating if you sneeze or cough. To lessen the effects of coughing or sneezing, grip onto this long, firm pillow that has a board in it and hold it against your chest. It will support your chest and reduce pain by softening the sneeze or cough when it happens." I kept this pillow on the side of my bed in case I needed it quickly at any time.

Throughout the day, I drifted in and out of sleep. Later that night, the nurses informed me that it was time to get out of bed and walk to the doorway leading to the hallway. I could not bend my body to get in and out of bed, and I could not use my arms to push myself out of bed or to lower myself into it, and no one could pull my arms to move me. I relied on the hospital aides and nurses to assist me once I was seated, making sure I didn't remove any tubes or harm myself or my sensitive body parts in the process. My chest didn't hurt when I used my arms by accident, so I continually reminded myself to keep them still. The aides wrapped their arms around my waist and hoisted me up. While I felt little pain, it was mentally exhausting. Sluggish and reluctant to walk, I knew it was necessary.

Once I was up, I used a walker and forced myself to walk. It felt like the walk was miles and miles through thick mud because it was enormously tough to make myself move. Putting one foot in front of the other was a challenge. Nurses surrounded me in case I fell, and one had a wheelchair behind me in case I needed to sit.

As we walked the short distance, I hunched over with all the tubes emerging from my torso, afraid they would come out if I straightened up. My family watched but I couldn't see them, as I kept my eyes focused on my hands gripping the sides of the walker or the floor and my blue hospital socks. Once I reached the threshold of the door I turned around slowly and made my way back to the room, where I sat in a chair instead of returning to bed. I was able to sit there for an hour as I spoke to my family; they were excited I accomplished my walking feat so soon after the surgery. The doctors were pleased with my progress, and I knew that the hard work of recovery had officially begun.

Chest Bubbles

A nursing student gave me a sponge bath in my bed early on Friday morning. I kept my eyes closed tightly shut as she washed my chest and abdomen, not wanting to see my body until I had to. The warm, soapy water felt good, but also terrible because my body was extremely sensitive to touch and everywhere she cleaned with the washcloth hurt. Although she was gentle, I wanted it to be over because of my hypersensitivity to everything.

As the anesthesia wore off, my arms ached with pain. Deep bruises from the implanted IV lines had left them dark blue and purple, but the ache was not from that. The pain was present all along my lower arm, from the wrist to the elbow. It was a tricky kind of ache to describe, not sharp but agonizing. While my fingers were pain-free, any movement of my arms felt miserable.

The pain in my arms wasn't the only unsettling feeling I was experiencing. On occasion, I could feel bubbles moving around in my lungs, like pop rocks bursting in my chest. Trained at an early age to report on everything going on in my body, I told Dr. Cole about this, and she responded, surprised, "You've always been so sensitive and aware. You feel everything. Most people never notice this stuff. I haven't had another patient complain about bubbles, but I don't doubt you." My chest bubbles continued as long as my tubes were in. It was uncomfortable but not unbearable.

Throughout the day, I was in and out of consciousness, feeling tired and unable to put up a facade of being perky. My head drooped and I lacked the strength to keep it upright when I sat up in bed or in a chair. Mom came to my aid and provided me with a black nylon neck pillow like the ones travelers use on planes, which helped me keep my head upright. I used it every day until I was strong enough to hold my neck up on my own.

My legs were in compression sleeves that inflated every so often to prevent blood clots forming from my lack of movement. A blood pressure cuff was constantly inflating on one arm, causing sharp pain along the bottom edges of the cuff that cut into my skin at every reading, which kept me awake. I had a catheter for urine and a needle of some kind in my neck that I did not ask about or look at.

Goodbye Chest Tubes and Hello PICC Line

The Saturday after the surgery was an eventful day. The doctors decided it was time to set up my PICC line, and the same afternoon they decided it was time to remove my chest tubes. A PICC line is a catheter that is used to administer medications and draw blood, which would free me from having to relive my childhood and adult distress about daily blood tests.

Owing to my nerves and memories from my chest tube removal at age six, the nurses felt I should have some antianxiety medication to get me through the procedure. I didn't want to take it since I wanted to be aware; I resisted, but they won, and I took the pill. As the medication started working and the nurses prepared to remove the tubes, the team responsible for administering the PICC line arrived. Since they were a team traveling around the hospital, their arrival time couldn't be scheduled. Therefore, they were given priority and began working on me before the chest tube removal.

The two-woman team in charge of the PICC line was considerate and friendly, patiently explaining everything they would do before proceeding. The antianxiety medication made me tired and I drifted in and out of consciousness as they installed the line in my upper arm. The numbing injection hurt, but other than that it went smoothly. The placement of the line in my upper arm was a relief, as the one remaining IV had not been staying in. The PICC line was hidden under the sleeve of my hospital gown and the tubes dangled behind me, providing me with a greater range of movement. Before I knew it, the procedure was over and it was time for the chest tubes to be removed.

Most of the antianxiety drug had worn off by the time everything was set up for removal. Dr. Washington's weekend physician's assistant (PA) strode confidently into the room. He had wild bushy hair and sneakers adorned with red lobsters that he made a point to show me. He reminded me of surgeons I had in the past, who didn't hear me or understand my anxieties. Although my parents tried to caution him how I might react, he paid them no attention. I faked laughing at his jokes in order not to cry or start screaming at him before he even started the procedure. My parents and Sam left the room so we could begin. I never saw what he did, but I felt everything.

He said smugly, "Yell and swear as much as you want to get through this," as I rolled my eyes knowing that wouldn't help at all. He opened my gown as I lay flat, keeping my eyes closed and felt cold, exposed in the air. As the stitches were removed, I didn't feel much and I was pretty quiet until the end. The last step of the process was pulling out the tubes. As he took them out, I could feel them pulling all the way up into my chest, being slowly yanked out without pausing. In reflex, my body jerked upward into a seated position as he pulled them out and I screamed and swore. I was crying and trying not to panic. When they were out, I fell back into a horizontal position in the bed, panting and crying as he cleaned up the area.

Then it was over. He left the room and I slept to try to forget about the trauma. Dr. Cole came to check in on me. She brought in an incentive spirometer/deep breathing exerciser, like one I remembered from childhood. I had to start using it now that the chest tubes were removed. *I'm not doing this with my full effort. I didn't when I was six either. It's so annoying and tedious even if it does something important.* Breathing in didn't hurt and I never pushed myself too far to the point of being uncomfortable. I just didn't like doing it or having an audience while I did it.

Sam reminded me every day to do my breathing exercises and watched me as I breathed in and out to make sure I complied. I advanced each day. Unlike when I was a child, I must have done a sufficient job using it as I didn't get pneumonia this second time around.

Daily Recovery Routine

After the chest tubes were removed, the hospital staff implemented a new daily routine. With the removal of the tubes, compression sleeves, urine catheter, and IV, I found myself able to move around with more ease and was getting out of bed more frequently. Every day at around 9 a.m., a nurse would come to my room and draw blood from my PICC line. I never felt or saw anything as she did this. She gave me my medications and helped me out of bed. I sat in the chair next to my bed to eat breakfast every day. While I ate, I watched everything going on in the hall. Usually, Sam would arrive during breakfast time and, after a brief visit, she would go to work for a few hours before returning in the afternoon. Mom would come to visit me around 9 or 10 a.m. and sometimes her visit would overlap with Sam's. During these visits, Mom and I would catch up on things she had missed. She would bring me cards from family and friends to read, which reminded me of the cards I received from my classmates when I was younger. Even though I didn't feel well, each card brought a smile to my face and motivated me to keep pushing through the hard times.

Lead doctors followed by a swarm of medical students no longer came to my bedside every morning to recite my condition specifics and poke at me. I think there must have been briefings in the hall so that when they came in, only a short exam was needed, along with a quick check-in to ask how I felt. After the morning examination by the doctors, Mom and I went on a daily walk on the hospital floor together, sometimes accompanied by a nurse to assist me. At first, I couldn't go far and tired easily, so I used a walker and shuffled slowly along, keeping my gaze fixed on the floor to avoid looking at the machines or things keeping me going. I had no interest in what was happening around me during the walk and focused only on walking as far as I had to before returning to my room. After my walk, I returned to bed for a nap. Later, I would wake up for lunch, and if there were tests like X-rays, I was wheeled away to other parts of the hospital. When I returned, Mom was waiting, and I would either take a nap or have a shower.

A few days after the surgery, I started taking daily showers in the bathing room located on the hospital floor. The nurse's aide and I entered the tiled room where there was a changing area with a seat. The aide wrapped my PICC line in a plastic bag to keep it dry during my shower and she undressed me in the changing area. I made sure to keep my eyes closed throughout the process. We would then walk slowly to the shower area, which was only a few steps away, where handheld shower nozzles were installed. While seated, I avoided looking at my upper body but did catch a glimpse of my thighs. *My legs are so big. My skin's shiny and taut from all this extra weight.* I weighed eleven pounds more since checking into the hospital because I had been pumped full of fluids. Along with all of my other medications, I took Lasix, a diuretic, to try to start losing the water weight I had gained. *I hope my thighs go back to normal soon.*

The aide assisted me in all aspects of taking a shower. She put shampoo in my hair and washed it because I couldn't raise my arms to do it myself. Additionally, she soaped my body and rinsed it off. She washed my chest and groin incisions every day to keep them clean. I usually became cold during the shower and shivered because only some parts of my body had warm water on them. *This is miserable but it's good to leave my room and get clean.*

Following my shower and nap, I would wake up to find Mom seated across from me, near the whiteboard, engrossed in a mystery novel. Her long artistic earrings changed daily, but her dependable presence remained constant. She would usually depart shortly thereafter, and Dad would arrive. In the late afternoon, Sam would stop by for her second visit. Depending on how I was feeling that day, I would walk a short distance down the hall or around the floor with Dad and Sam. Sometimes, we would sit in the solarium, which was located at the opposite end of the hallway from my room, beyond the nurses' desk. Afterward, we would return to my room, since my dinner was usually delivered around 5:30 p.m.

Sam and Dad often left the hospital to get takeout dinner for themselves so we could eat together in my room. While they were out, I would usually take a nap after our walk, as it was quite tiring for me. Upon their return, I would listen to them talk about their outing. Early on during my hospital stay there was a Red Sox event in a nearby park, and they brought me back balloon animals, Red Sox signs, and a baseball-shaped stress ball. I came to rely on the ball. Every time I had to undergo a test or needed something to take my anger out on or take my mind off my pain and anxiety, I would squeeze it. After dinner, my family would leave for the day and I would go to sleep. If I struggled to fall asleep during the night, I would count down the hours until my first visitors would arrive in the morning.

As the days went by in the hospital, my doctors said I was doing well. I was experiencing less pain with each passing day.

Mom offered me her phone in case I wanted to browse any websites or talk to anyone, but that had no appeal. I didn't want to email or talk with my friends or have any visitors outside of my family, just as I hadn't wanted to when I was six years old. Over time, I slowly took interest in the outside world. I felt like looking at a nail polish blog I liked. It was a small step, but it was the first time that I had taken notice of life going on outside of the hospital that my family hadn't told me about.

Every morning I received a menu to choose my food options for the day, including breakfast for the following day. My food was not restricted, other than limiting sodium, so there were many options to choose from. Some might think hospital food is unappealing, but I usually like the range of options and enjoy not cooking for myself. To add some excitement to my meals, Sam and I started a game where she would choose my meals as a surprise. I eagerly awaited the reveal every time. Most days I had a spaghetti lunch (one of my favorite meals) with surprise side dishes and varied drinks, and I always had a mystery entrée at dinner—sometimes spaghetti again.

Phoebe

After six days of this, August 15th arrived. It was a much-anticipated day because I had a one-of-a-kind visitor. Sam worked with the nurses and volunteer office to arrange for a therapy dog to come and visit me. Her determination and planning paid off. I have always felt a unique connection with animals that aid the sick, knowing how much their attention means to someone who doesn't feel their best. Both my parents and Sam promptly arrived in the morning all together for the first time during my hospital stay. We all impatiently awaited the dog's arrival, not knowing what to expect.

Therapy dogs did not routinely visit the cardiac floor, so it was an unusual sight for the medical staff and patients alike when the dog finally arrived. We heard many people excitedly saying "A dog!" as she passed their rooms and walked to the end of the hallway to my room. Sam and I looked at each other with enormous smiles on our faces when we heard the chorus announcing her arrival. We could hear toenails tapping down the hall and tags jangling like Christmas bells. Suddenly, a large, light-colored golden retriever lumbered into my room with her owner.

"This is Phoebe!" Her owner proudly introduced us as she climbed into my bed and lay next to me, panting. I was interested, but not as engaged as I usually am with animals. Because of the pain in my arms, I couldn't pet her in the way I would have liked, although I appreciated having her in my bed and stroked her long, silky hair the best I could. *Such an official vest. Her body's so warm on my leg.*

My family interacted with her more than I did and they spoke with her owner at great length, inquiring about Phoebe and the work she does. Crowds of nurses watched at the door and came in and out to pet Phoebe. I offered Phoebe my stress baseball to play with, but she wasn't interested. She was more of a sit-and-be-patted kind of dog. The visit helped pick up all of our spirits immensely.

Two Mysteries Explained

My arm pain still persisted after the surgery. I mentioned it to all of my doctors and nurses because I was so uncomfortable, and no one could explain it. The ache never let up, and even simple movements like brushing my teeth hurt. I pushed through it rather than take more medication. Doctors offered me narcotics to help, but I refused to take them because I didn't want to feel tired and drugged anymore, having stopped taking narcotics a few days earlier. *I remember this pain! It happened after the ablations but for only a day or so. But why? When will it stop?*

After Phoebe's visit, Dr. Anderson (my cardiologist prior to Dr. Cole) came in to examine me. I hadn't seen her for many years, but

I always knew she was updated on my status. She listened when I described the agony from my arm pain, and she diagnosed it.

"It's nerve pain from when your arms were held down on the table during the surgery. I experienced this pain myself after surgery. This surgery took much longer than your ablations did, which is why your arms are still hurting," she said. "I'll arrange for a physical therapist to come see you to try to help."

Dr. Anderson also arranged for me to receive a care bag made by family members of patients with cardiac conditions. Inside the canvas bag were general toiletries. It made the hospital feel like a hotel with amenities. Throughout my stay in the hospital, I noticed that my sense of smell was extremely heightened, and I could smell even the tiniest odors very strongly. Body odors and food smells, in particular, were potent. I didn't mention this sensitivity to anyone as it didn't seem significant.

I did, however, tell the nurses I was nauseated. I experienced daily, continuous nausea and the nurses gave me injections of antinausea medication even though they weren't sure why I felt this way. The medication made me tired and I would fall asleep. When I woke up, the sickness remained, but I never vomited. I went through the care bag smelling the new shampoos and conditioners and didn't feel nauseated. *Of course! It's the hospital shampoo making me sick!* After every shower, I always felt the queasiest, reacting to my heightened sense of smell. I had all of the hospital shampoos in my room thrown away and I instantly was on the mend.

Last Evening and Discharge from the Hospital

On August 15th, the same day we met Phoebe, Sam and Dad went out to pick up their food for dinner as usual. They brought it back to my room to eat. I watched with envy as they took bites out of the clear plastic takeout containers of the creamy-yellow chicken salad with raisins, carrots, and spices. The smell made my mouth water for the first time since I was in the hospital. They normally offered me some of their dinner every night and I refused, but that night I ate a couple of bites. It was my first taste of nonhospital food in a week. The aromatic smells of trips past and the taste of chicken bursting with hot flavor were too hard to resist. Sam joked as I chewed the chicken, slowly savoring it, "Seeing Phoebe has woken something up inside of you!" I laughed in agreement and they went home after dinner.

My roommate's TV played a Lady Gaga song, and I sang along and danced a little while lying in bed before falling asleep. Just a few hours earlier, I had little interest in anything going on in the outside world and had always ignored the constant blaring of my roommate's television, which was on twenty-four hours a day. I never turned my own TV on during my entire hospital stay, which was unlike me. I wanted to have as much quiet as possible to focus on my daily tasks. Being disconnected from everything meant I didn't feel I was missing out on anything or had to push myself to get better faster than I was ready for. That night, I had vivid dreams and heavy sweating, and it seemed like all the anesthesia and medication was leaving my body.

I woke up clearheaded on Wednesday, seven days after the surgery. I sat up in my bed and waited to see the PA I liked speaking with. He had tried to help me with my concerns and also took an interest in learning about my heart condition, so we had spent extra time together talking during my admission. When he came down the hall and saw me sitting up, he came right in.

I blurted out, "I sweated a lot; I want a shower and I want to go home!"

He gave me the once-over and said, "I see the difference in you. I'll confer with Dr. Washington after checking your daily blood test results and see if you can go home."

While I waited for information, I moved to sit in the chair near my bed. My breakfast tray arrived, and for the first time, I thought, *I don't like this food. The bagel tastes like stale cardboard. The cream cheese can't disguise it. The juice is too sweet.* It was a real sign I was ready to leave.

When Sam arrived, I pretended to feel unwell, and I faked being asleep while sitting in my chair. Then I lifted my head and said with wide eyes, "Guess what? I might go home today!" Surprised and excited, we waited for the PA to return with an update. A while later he returned as I was taking my morning walk in the hallway with Sam.

He said, "Everyone agrees you can go home as long as you can show me you can run to the nurse's station at the end of the hall." He was kidding of course and merely wanted me to continue my morning walk, but I told him I could do it. I gathered up my hospital gown so I wouldn't trip and ran to the station.

Not running quickly or gracefully at all, I'm sure I looked crazy. Hunching over, as the leads from my heart monitor always pulled my chest down, I ran slowly in a bent position. It felt like my chest was heavy and I had labored breathing. *This isn't as easy as I thought it'd be. But I'm not going to stop and show them that I'm defeated.* Movement around me stopped as everyone watched in the hall and at the nurses' desk, astonished as I passed them by.

Clapping and cheering abounded as I breathlessly went back to my room to rest. I sat in my chair and waited for my final body check. Sam left the room when the nurses came in. When they checked my body, one said the dreaded words ruining my earlier triumphant moment, "You still have a stitch in your stomach." This caught me completely off guard as I had kept my eyes closed during the check and I hadn't seen my body in the shower. After such a high from running down the hall, I couldn't feel any lower and began crying. The idea of going through another removal procedure was crushing. I was also angry that the PA who had performed the removal had missed this. *I can't go through another removal. That stupid PA missed it.* After feeling so strong and happy to go home, I now was back to square one, feeling weak and upset.

Open-heart surgery can heighten your emotions and cause you to cry over small problems and pains, and minor events can feel bigger than they actually are. *I'm going to have to take an antianxiety pill to relax. I don't want to feel groggy again from medication.* One nurse said, "I'll get the PA to come to check and give his opinion if it is a scab or stitch."

In the meantime, Sam returned to the room to find me crying in a chair. I told her what happened and we anxiously waited for the PA to come to my room. When he entered, he examined the area with a handheld light and said, "It's just a scab. If it does turn out to be a stitch, you can remove it yourself later at home."

Elated there were no more procedures, my tears stopped right away. *I'm in control. I can perform my own stitch removal and don't need to have another person touching me and bothering me.* Just as Sam left for work for a few hours, Mom arrived. I let her know I could return home and I had run down the hall. She called Dad to let him know the good news and to arrange my transportation home.

Mom and I went on a walk past the nurse's station where I happened to run into the physical therapist Dr. Anderson arranged to help me with my arm pain. He didn't fully examine me or provide a solution to my quandary, mostly because of my impending return home. Although discouraged, I was still glad to be going home and decided to wait out the arm pain to see if it would improve.

The final test I had to pass in order to go home was to walk up a full flight of stairs without any heartbeat irregularities. A nurse took me into the hospital stairway while another nurse monitored my EKG at the nurse's station. I could walk as slowly as I wanted, but I couldn't hold onto the railing to avoid pulling on it and hurting my sternum. The nurse stood behind me, ready to assist in case I became weak. Climbing up the stairs was like climbing a mountain. I could do it slowly, and it was demanding; nevertheless, determined to go home, I kept pushing myself up. At the top, I was out of breath, but I passed the test and felt no irregular beats. I was good to go.

When I returned to my room later, the head discharge nurse gave Mom and me detailed directions in a nineteen-page packet on how to care for myself at home. We went through the directions, which included information about daily care, instructions for bathing and cleaning my incisions, and activity restrictions such as not lifting more than a couple of pounds, not pushing or pulling with my arms, not lifting my arms overhead to do things like washing my hair, and not driving for at least four to six weeks.

My medication schedule and directions for home were even more complicated than the average instructions for postsurgical care because I was on the blood thinner Coumadin. The packet contained detailed instructions on how to take the pill, the restrictions it imposed, and possible side effects. My blood needed to be tested frequently to make sure I had the right medication levels, which I detested. I also had to monitor my intake of leafy greens because they could interfere with the blood thinner's effectiveness.

I met with the special Coumadin nurse, Anne, ahead of discharge. She was assigned to help me regulate my levels and handle any issues that might arise. Anne told me, "I'll let you know the days you have to go to the hospital for testing and will call you as soon as the results are in. If your levels demand it, you'll have to adjust your leafy green intake and your medication dose."

I bobbed my head in agreement, listening to everything she said. *I won't have to do this for long. Dr. Washington said I won't have to keep taking Coumadin after our first postop appointment in six weeks. That day can't come soon enough.*

After Anne left, I had one last X-ray and then my PICC line was removed, causing a momentary sting. I dressed but found I couldn't button the shorts I had worn a week ago when checking into the hospital because of all the weight I had gained from being pumped full of fluids and medications. Doctors expected my weight to go down from medications they sent me home with and time would help, so I tried not to dwell on it. With Mom's assistance, I removed my baseball decorations and photos of Sam's dog from the wall and packed my belongings. Dad arrived with Sam to take me home. An aide with a wheelchair appeared and it was time to go. It all happened quickly, but I made sure to leave my hospital identification bracelet on the bed poignantly and got into the wheelchair.

My parents, Sam, and I went down the hall as the aide wheeled me. I smiled and said goodbye to the nurses at the station and then we went down to the main lobby. *It's all too much. The nurses and aides can't help me anymore. I won't have an adjustable bed and no one can help me in the bathroom. Everything went so fast. It doesn't feel real that I even had the surgery. I don't feel stronger, I feel weak and heavy from all this weight.* I started to cry, and Sam tried to talk to me except I couldn't respond, and Mom told her to let me be as I sat staring out the large windows onto the main hospital driveway.

Dad pulled up, and I was pushed in a wheelchair to the car, and we drove back to my parents' house. When we arrived, Sam had made me a sign from a printout of a photo of her chihuahua/ Jack Russell terrier, Josie, welcoming me home. Her bright black eyes, which could melt the coldest ice, shone through the photo like a smile. Slowly, I walked up the front walkway, climbed up the stairs to the sign, and happily entered the house. There, I sat in a chair, feeling exhausted. My family fussed over me, making sure I was comfortable and had my medications.

After a short wait, Sam and Josie arrived. Josie was happy to see me after my long absence. She is about eleven pounds and likes to sit in laps. Upon our reunion, wagging her tail furiously, she flew into my lap and landed right on my groin incisions. The pain was blinding and burning. Tears sprung to my eyes, but I didn't complain. I closed my eyes and squeezed my baseball stress ball until the pain lessened. Worried the incisions might have opened, I searched my shorts, but I didn't see any red marks. I patted Josie's white-and-brown spotted back, and rubbed her brown-and-white striped ear, feeling better after a while. From then on, I kept a pillow on my lap so she'd land on the pillow instead of my legs.

In addition to bringing Josie, Sam brought me homemade peanut butter cookies to eat. *Just like Grandma made.* These cookies were larger, but the recipe was the same, with crisscross patterns from the fork indentations on the top.

Recovery at Home

My first night at home was rough. My bed was not adjustable, so I needed a triangle-shaped wedge pillow to prevent my chest from feeling crushed while lying down. The inability to change positions resulted in soreness, making it hard for me to sleep. During the first full day at home during recovery, I sat in a chair in the front room of the house to watch the day go by. Holding my head up was still challenging, and I continued to use an airplane neck pillow to maintain an upright posture in chairs. Feeling tired, I snacked on deviled eggs Mom had prepared for me while waiting for my pain medication to take effect.

As I couldn't raise my arms to put on shirts, I had to wear a new wardrobe of button-up tops and larger bras. My previous bras were now too tight owing to the chest swelling. Mom had gone out to buy me bras without underwire, which were kept closed by an elastic string attached in the back, tied like a bikini, since I was too big to use the default clasps. In addition, I wore baggy shorts to relieve pressure from my groin incisions and slip-on shoes since I couldn't bend down to tie laces.

To flush the toilet, I used a grabber to push the lever, since I was incapable of leaning over to press it myself. The pain in my arms persisted, and Mom had an idea to help alleviate it. She placed the gel wrist rest from her computer keyboard under my arm, and it was the first thing that brought me any relief. I alternated its placement from under one arm to the other, and it worked for a short period of time.

Dr. Cole assigned me homework to walk every day as a part of my recovery. There were ups and downs each day of my recovery and some days I could do more than others. Sometimes I walked in the neighborhood to see my dog friends and sometimes I walked in new places. I walked around the makeup counters of a department store at the mall to get accustomed to crowds again and picked up a new lip gloss along the way. On another day, I walked around town to get a sandwich for lunch. Every day, I walked somewhere new, trying to keep it interesting and nonrepetitive.

Feeling overwhelmed by the outside stimulation that TV provided, I needed alternative ways to keep myself entertained. Luckily, Sam came over every day before work and brought Josie with her to keep me company. After getting an estimate of Josie's arrival time, I'd slowly walk from my bedroom to the foyer to open the front door and eagerly await her arrival. As soon as she bounded into the house, I couldn't help but smile as she excitedly ran over to me. I couldn't bend down to pet her, but I would sit on the couch, and she would jump up and shower me with joyful kisses. *I'm glad Josie's here to keep me company and entertain me. Josie's all I need to feel like I'm not missing out on anything by spending all day resting.* She joined Dad and me on walks and we'd show her the neighborhood trees and creatures. Because Sam brought Josie over every day, I saw Sam more frequently than previously in our adult lives. When she came to pick Josie up at the end of her workday, we'd catch up. *It feels like when I was living at home after college again.* I became used to my recovery routine and my family's care.

I grew more comfortable with Sam as my caregiver, and I began to display how it truly felt when I was sick. She handled it well, but one thing sticks with me. I was not allowed to sit in the front seat of a car in case the airbags went off and hurt my sternum.

This restriction didn't bother me at all. Sam told me, "It's upsetting that you're too fragile to sit in the front seat." Taken aback, I reconsidered how situations that seemed normal or acceptable to me could be troubling to others. It was hard to hear she was dismayed over something I thought was trivial. I've come to take small things to be big and big things to be small.

Sam said, "You always complain about the little things like scars, and not what actually matters like having had open-heart surgery!"

I didn't say anything, but I thought, *the surgery's over, but the scars are forever.*

After leaving the hospital, I was unable to manage my complicated medication regimen on my own. Remembering all the types of medications, times, and doses was too much for me. To help me with this, Dad created a chart on the computer that listed everything in detail, including the medication schedule. He printed it out and kept it on the desk in my room, allowing me to keep track of everything easily. This chart reminded me of the childhood journal Dad made for himself and had shared with me. It also tracked my daily progress, detailing my walks, and was a nice thing to look back on after my recovery to see how far I had come.

I cleaned my incisions with a washcloth and soap during my daily showers, which I found to be a calming ritual. I looked forward to it every day. Prior to bathing, I examined some parts of my body in the mirror. I avoided looking at my chest since I wasn't ready to see my scar, which was still covered by surgical tape. Instead, I noticed the raw skin on my neck resulting from the needle removal a few days earlier. *This better not leave a scar.* I also found sticky tape residue left over from procedures all over my body, exposed as clothing rubbed on it and left behind glue with lint stuck in it. I diligently rubbed this glue off whenever I found it and kept searching until I was sure all of it was gone.

Coumadin Testing

Two days after my discharge from the hospital, I returned to MGH for my first Coumadin blood test. *I hope this works this first time and doesn't hurt too much.* When my parents and I arrived at the hospital, I rode in a wheelchair to the blood lab as I wasn't strong enough to walk far. Mom left to park the car and I felt pathetic being wheeled around by Dad. My head drooped in the chair, and I didn't make eye contact with anyone. *I feel gross in these baggy clothes. I'm fat and weak. I hope I don't know anyone here.* I looked around the waiting room and names were loudly called to enter the lab. Dad stayed in the waiting room when I was taken back by a technician for the blood test.

Finger pricks won't be so bad. They weren't before in the hospital years ago. The technician did the test and it hurt terribly. I don't know if it was because I was already weak or it really is that bad, but it felt like the needle went right into my bone. Tears started and I tried to keep smiling even though it hurt so much and the technician apologized and rubbed my finger. The technician filled her vials and then wheeled me back out to Dad, and we went into the elevator. I told him how much the test hurt, showing him my bandaged finger and he surprised me by saying merrily, "We're going to the gift shop!" My mood brightened, but I still held tightly onto my hurt finger.

When I was six, after my first surgery while I was staying in the hospital, I was wheeled down to the gift shop where Dad bought me a flower. I could pick any flower I wanted and I chose a yellow rose. This time around during my hospital stay, Dad asked a nurse if we could go down to the gift shop, but they refused because new rules stated that patients couldn't leave the floor. I was frustrated about not being able to follow the same routine as my first surgery, but this special trip made up for it.

As Dad wheeled me to the cool refrigerator at the back of the shop, I saw through the glass doors many bouquets but no single flowers like my yellow rose. We waited for someone to help us, and once they did, they let me choose one flower out of any bouquet I wanted. I chose a purple-and-white calla lily and Dad surprised me with a helium balloon. The balloon had a picture of a dog like Josie that said, "Feeling ruff? Get well soon." *Just like when I was little, I have a balloon and a flower. My finger hurts less.*

When we returned home, another surprise was waiting. A delivery of a bouquet of flowers was waiting outside the front door. Charlie, my British friend, who was living in Munich, had a local florist send flowers to me as a surprise while I was recovering at home. It was comforting to have it, as my finger still hurt and did for over a week from the blood test. Seeing and smelling the flower from Dad and the bouquet of roses made me feel better.

At home after my blood test, the Coumadin nurse, Anne, called me to discuss the results. "I want you to adjust your pills and leafy greens for the week to try to get your levels as perfect as they can be."

"Fine," I replied, "But I want to make a change to my future blood tests. The finger prick was unbearable. I'd rather go to the MGH satellite location where I can have blood draws rather than finger pricks."

Anne agreed, since it made no difference to her. After the first experience, I went to have my blood tested five more times. Anne always called shortly after the tests with updates, sometimes as the car was pulling into the garage after our twenty-minute drive. *These blood tests are taking over my life. It's so irritating. I hate changing my food, too, and I don't think I could balance my diet without Mom. I made the right choice about the valve type. If I'd gotten the mechanical valve I'd be at the hospital all the time. This will end soon enough; I can do this for a while longer.*

Hope

Choosing to take the easier path used to be my modus operandi. Stairs and hills were challenging for me. In the past, I avoided them whenever possible, choosing to take escalators and elevators when they were available, and planned my walking routes around them. When I saw a hill or stairs I always unconsciously determined if I could tackle them or not. When I was younger, my parents planned my activities to dodge inclines altogether. When I went on walks with family and peers, they went much faster than me and I fell behind. I ended up walking alone, as rushing to keep up made me tired. I found that this allowed me to better appreciate my surroundings. On a walk someone once said to me, "You're always aware of everything, so observant." I often heard rustling leaves of nearby creatures and spotted animals on the ground, such as inchworms slowly crossing the road. I took the time to watch the tiny green worms arching their bodies to cross the dauntingly large sidewalk. Their presence made me feel less alone, especially when everyone else walked further ahead of me.

While I was recovering, I found that going up the steep wooden stairs from my parents' backyard onto the deck was less difficult than before. Previously, these stairs had been somewhat challenging for me, but after experiencing AFib, they became even more arduous. Ten days after my surgery, however, I climbed up these stairs and noticed that I was no longer as out of breath at the top as I used to be. The same was true when I climbed the stairs from the basement to the first floor in my parents' house.

I began to experiment with my stamina when I left home to see what I could do and to find out if anything had indeed changed. In my parents' neighborhood, there is a long, steep street with houses on both sides with large grassy yards. Before the surgery, I could walk up this hill slowly, taking a short rest on the way up. I never went up this street by choice on walks. When Mom and I went on a walk shortly after my return home from the hospital, I asked, "Can we go up the hill?" *I think I can do it, since I climbed the deck and basement stairs.*

"No, I don't think that's a good idea."

We didn't do it because she was used to limiting my activities and being cautious. About two weeks after the surgery, Dad went on a walk with me, and I asked him if I could go up the hill. He agreed and we started up it. *This feels different already! I'm breathing normally. I don't need a rest at the halfway point.* Taking the same-sized strides and going the same pace as always, it was easier. One house away from the top of the hill where I usually took a rest and looked at my neighbors' zip line, I journeyed on without stopping. Once I reached the top, I wasn't exhausted. *I made it so fast, and before Dad!* We were both surprised and eagerly told Mom and Sam this major news. I didn't want to become overly excited in case I couldn't do it again as I was used to so much disappointment; but I repeated this feat a couple of days later. *Life might be changing ...*

Around this time, I began comparing myself to the character Benjamin Button from the short story "The Curious Case of Benjamin Button" by F. Scott Fitzgerald. Benjamin ages in reverse and experiences new abilities as he becomes younger and younger. I wasn't becoming younger, but I was experiencing new abilities people have been able to do since they were young and take for granted. *Appreciate it, it might not last,* I reminded myself.

The Scar Reveal

Approximately two and half weeks after the surgery at the end of August, it was time to remove the tape on my chest incision. Individual pieces of clear plastic adhesive strips of tape went horizontally across my chest, each about two inches long. The tape peeled up at the ends somewhat each day and a few pieces fell off naturally on their own. Since they were clear, I saw my scar a little bit, but I had not thoroughly looked at it.

Feeling frightened, I knew it was time to take off the tape. Without any excuse for delay, I chose to do the removal while taking a shower. I left the bathroom door open so I could shout for Mom in case I needed her to come in. Moving slowly, putting off the removal for as long as possible, I turned on the faucet, waited for the water to warm up, and climbed over the tub railing into the shower. I wet my hair and let my skin become damp to help ease some of the tape removal. I slowly peeled one piece of tape off at a time. With one hand I held the tape, and with the other I held the skin beneath it taut. Some strips were tightly attached to my skin, but others came right off without any pulling or stickiness. When I removed them, I closed my eyes and pulled them up slowly, squealing as I did it. It didn't hurt; it was more a feeling of discomfort as my skin raised up. I eventually removed all of the tape and saw my scar for the first time when I stepped out of the shower and looked into the steamy mirror, glad the view was not one hundred percent clear.

My new scar was bright red and purple and, surprisingly, it was longer than my original scar. My first scar ended inside the area where a bra band covers the torso. Now the scar would be exposed underneath the bottom of a bra or bikini top. I resented it. *It's now double the width. Dr. Washington said it would be on top of the old one. It's not! Now they are side-by-side. The same with the chest-tube scars. There are new red marks above the old white scars. It's doubled, too. And there are some raised parts in the middle. I guess a V-neck shirt won't show the raised parts, but I can't hide it in a bathing suit.* I couldn't bear to look at my body. I cried and kept my eyes facing up so I couldn't see anything anymore. I thought about my friend's advice, "Own it." But I didn't have the confidence yet. *Is this gonna be a problem with a boyfriend?*

I knew the new low-cut shirts I had bought on a whim prior to the surgery would remain at the back of my closet for years to come. The day-to-day matter of wanting to cover my scar had an impact on my psyche in ways struggling on stairs did not, and it persists today. My scar will never go away, while stairs are merely a temporary problem.

I put on my button-up shirt and kept it open, calling Mom into the room. "Look at it: it's hideous! It's not flat anymore," I cried.

Mom looked at my chest, "It will get better as it heals. It's just swelling," she said.

I tried to believe her as I buttoned my shirt, but I had my doubts.

As time went on, the red and purple faded, becoming paler, but other than that, nothing much changed. *I don't want anyone to see it.* It's a massive change I have to get used to and maybe, with time, I will become more comfortable with it.

Venturing Outside, Back to the Healthy World, and Seeing Friends

When a person falls ill, it feels like time stops. The world continues to move forward without them, but they are unable to engage. They may be in the hospital, away from home, or absent from work, school, and their usual activities. It's similar to being stopped at a traffic light at an intersection, where you see surrounding cars moving on with their drivers living their lives. Although you might want to step on the gas and go, you can't until it's your turn and it's safe to do so.

To focus on healing, it's easier for me not to think about my outside life and what I might be missing. Once I started to recover, I needed to find out what I had missed. The transition was not easy because I had to take an interest in others after all the attention was on me and my recovery. It can be hard to go back and, as Mabel says, "It's okay to have a return-to-life meltdown."

It took me a while to be ready to start emailing and seeing people again. After some days at home, I decided I was ready to start reconnecting with people. Taking out my phone, I caught up on emails and texts. Visitors started coming over to my parents' house to see me. I enjoyed talking with them, learning about what they had been doing during the last month. I answered questions about myself but tried not to draw much attention to what I had been through, not wanting to dwell on it. I also began catching up on TV shows. Since I had two more months off from work, I had plenty of time to gradually get back to my normal routine. I didn't have to rush anything and could enjoy events as they came up during my recovery process.

One important event in August was Sam's thirtieth birthday. We had celebrated our milestone birthdays in July in Vermont, but her actual birthday is in August. I had asked Dr. Washington during our office visit, "Will I be up to going out to eat to celebrate Sam's birthday at the end of the month? It'll be about three weeks after the surgery."

He smiled and nodded, assuring me, "You'll be well enough to have a good time and probably up to doing more than you think you'll be able to. You might not have the energy to celebrate for long, but you'll be an active participant."

On the big day, my family and I went out for a celebratory sushi lunch. Little by little, I progressed along the sidewalk in the summer heat to the restaurant and sat down inside for the meal. I enjoyed eating the sushi Sam ordered for the table, the warm and crispy gyoza, and white rice. After a while talking and eating, I grew tired from sitting for such a long time. My family understood, and since we had finished eating it was no problem to return home. I had taken another step in reentering the healthy world.

The next day a funny coincidence occurred between my first surgery at age six and my second at age thirty-five. While recovering from my second surgery, I found myself in the garden with Dad, helping him with weeding. I pulled out weeds with my toes because I could not bend over. I found out later, after reading Dad's diary from my first recovery, I had helped garden then, too, by planting flowers.

Another time when events seemed to come full circle was on August 21st. A rare solar eclipse occurred, visible across the United States. While in the hospital, family friends had sent me a card with eclipse-viewing glasses, so I was excited when the time came and I got to wear them. I brought a stool outside to sit on to watch the eclipse with my parents and Josie. Glad to be out of work, I could watch it outside for a long time with no other commitments taking away from my enjoyment of it. *This is like when I was in middle school.* I've never enjoyed school, and twice a year I missed a day of school to attend my cardiologist appointments in downtown Boston. On one of these appointment days when everyone else was stuck inside at school, Mom and I witnessed a solar eclipse, just like we did in 2017.

Turning a Corner

For a couple of days in August, I felt some flutters. *What's that? I've lost more sensitivity. It's AFib, right? But what if it's not? I've been doing so well. I don't know what's going on inside of me!* Aware of every little bodily event, I took my pulse several times throughout the day. Unsure of what was going on, I called Dr. Cole. She didn't think the flutters were AFib, but she suggested an EKG to be sure, which found my heart to be in normal rhythm. The flutters were probably my heart adjusting to everything. I felt all right otherwise overall and I was still doing well after this one hiccup.

Four days after my EKG, I had my first office checkup with Dr. Cole since the surgery. She confirmed what I already knew and sensed; everything was great. There was nothing of note on my EKG and I was healing properly. Dr. Cole read more results and said to me, "You have to keep walking every day to keep strengthening your heart. Would you like to start cardiac rehab?"

Not knowing what people did there, I didn't know if it was something I could do. I looked at her in confusion awaiting more explanation. She explained, "I want you to start attending rehab to ease back into exercise while being monitored in a safe environment in case anything goes wrong. Once you start, if you don't like it, you can quit." She placed me on the waitlist for a spot to open up in several weeks' time and told me to expect a call when I could go.

The new exercise program might be fun. Leaving the appointment, I felt hungry. *My taste's different now. I've been starving for white rice and the taste of alcohol ever since Sam's birthday party. I want it all the time now. Drinking can make my heart beat irregularly, but I want a drink.* I merely wanted the flavor of alcohol but never the intoxicated feeling going along with it, so I drank small amounts. *Root beer and mustard don't taste good anymore. Now they're too sour. I don't know why my taste buds have changed.*

By the end of August, I noticed progress in different areas. My weight finally returned to its before-surgery level, which allowed me to discontinue some of my medications. This made life less complicated for both me and my parents. Although my arms continued to ache, it was a consistent and unchanging discomfort that I had become accustomed to. My walks stretched longer distances from walks on the town bike path, around the local farmers market, and to a nearby bakery.

I continued to work on becoming stronger as I had a momentous day to look forward to on September 1st. I had tickets to the Lady Gaga concert at Fenway Park. Ahead of the show, my family urged me to rest and get ready for the day so I could fully enjoy the concert. Little did I know, another surprise was booked for that day.

Blueberry and Maxi

For many years on Facebook, I followed two therapy dog pages, Blueberry and her friend, Maximus. Both dogs were pit bulls, short, with compact muscles, around seventy to eighty pounds. Blueberry was gray and Maxi was tan colored. Blueberry and Maxi visited people who were ill or had experienced trauma. I loved to read their stories about visiting patients and comforting people. Their stories were the highlight of my day.

Whenever I had cardioversions and procedures, in the waiting room, I always asked Mom in a joking manner, "Am I sick enough to meet Blueberry?"

"No," she'd sigh. "Blueberry's needed elsewhere, with sicker people."

Blueberry was known for visiting people in hospice and nursing homes, as well as providing comfort after terrorist events. Hospitals were not a common place for her to visit. Maxi also visited similar places, but not as frequently as Blueberry did. Prior to my surgery, Sam asked me about my wishes if the surgery was successful. I told her I wanted to meet Blueberry.

On the morning of September 1st, I got dressed as usual in my button-up shirt and baggy jeans. I prepared to go on my daily walk with Dad when my family convinced me to go outside with them instead. *OH MY GOSH! Blueberry and Maxi are in the driveway! I can't believe it. My favorite dogs in the entire world are here to see me!* I instantly dropped to my knees and smothered them with hugs and kisses, petting their warm and soft fur. They kissed me back and wagged their tails, extremely well behaved while wearing their working vests.

Their owners, my family, and I took the dogs into the basement of my house to play and to get to know one another. *I love them even more in person. Their moms are so kind and generous.* I cuddled and petted both dogs as long as I wanted, and the dogs never tried to get away from me to do something else. Their owners made sure they were gentle and never did more than I could handle and kept them off of my chest. The dogs not only played with me but also with my parents and Sam.

In the warm weather we took the dogs into the backyard and took off their service vests so they would know they were "off the clock" and could do whatever they pleased. In the fenced yard, they ran free and I ran a small amount, at a slow pace, with them. I sprinkled treats around the yard to get them to run after me. We played fetch with sticks and catch with tennis balls. *I'm free, like them! This feels like a dream. They're choosing me without being told to. They must like me.* Blueberry put her paw on my arm and Maxi shook hands. *Today feels magical.*

We took pictures and videos to capture all of the fun we had together during the visit. A while later they returned home. Blueberry and Maxi made all the hardship worth it. They gave me emotional strength to continue my recovery. Whenever I was anxious, I thought of them and I instantly felt gratitude for all I was going through, since it meant I got to meet them.

Lady Gaga and Hair Dye

After meeting Blueberry and Maxi, I went to the Lady Gaga concert at Fenway Park. My ticket had been purchased several months before I knew the surgery was happening, and I was determined to make it there during my recovery. I had not ventured into downtown Boston, aside from the hospital, or been around large crowds since going to work in July. My worries about people knocking into me and hurting my chest deterred me from crowded places. A friend who worked at Fenway Park arranged for me to watch the concert with her in the press box away from the people on the field. We could hear the music and see everything in a less crowded, enclosed space from the indoor room above home plate with huge glass windows that were wide open. Lady Gaga's strong voice filled the room and her sparkly costumes shone in the setting sun. Taking pictures of the best outfits, I also studied all the details with my binoculars. We sat in seats in front of the large open windows and I stood up to sing my favorite songs. The old me from before AFib came back as I danced. I wasn't totally myself yet or back to having high energy levels, but walking a far distance from the car to the seats, dancing, and staying out late wasn't as exhausting as I expected it to be.

The concert marked a turning point in my recovery when I regained some of my independence. I began to do more for myself like cooking some meals. Some days my energy levels fluctuated, but I was walking more. Two days after the concert, I went over to Sam's apartment for dinner without my parents. I hadn't really left my parents' house and hadn't been away from them except for the concert, still getting used to life after the surgery.

While I lay on the couch after dinner Sam asked me, "What do you want to do with the rest of your time off from work? You're doing so well."

We realized around then in my recovery I was not as tired and feeble as we had thought I would be. *This might be my one time when I've got so much time off from work with no other responsibilities than taking care of myself. I should take advantage of this.* I confidently stated, "I want to dye my hair blue!" *My office would never allow this.*

"Let's do it!" Sam enthusiastically grabbed her car keys and we went to the store.

On the drive, I emailed Dr. Washington, "Can I dye my hair? I'm not sure what will happen if it gets into my incision. Also, yesterday, my last chest tube scab fell off and I noticed a stitch inside of me." *I don't want to go to the hospital to take the stitch out. I want an answer and for this to be over.* "Do I have to come in to have it removed?"

Dr. Washington responded instantly, "The dye's fine. You can take the stitch out yourself."

Great! I'll be able to control this. I won't have to have any more procedures if I do it right.

Sam and I arrived at the store and went to the hair-dye aisle. I breezed past the conventional blonde, brown, and black looks straight to the rainbow of colors in the temporary dye section. After careful consideration and consultation with Sam, we settled on a teal blue and returned home.

First, I dealt with the stitch. Standing at the bathroom sink, I was ready to confront the removal. Like an army captain about to go into battle, I faced something terrifying. I lay my instruments out on a towel on the sink counter and took a deep breath. I washed my hands, put alcohol on the scissors, kept some tissues nearby in case I bled and left the door open a crack in case I needed to yell for Sam to come in to help me. Gripping the thread, I closed my eyes, took another deep breath, and pulled out the black stitch. *This feels like nothing. Just some pulling inside.* There was a tiny dot of blood on my tissue, but nothing disturbing. *It's over and it was so simple. Time to dye my hair. I wish I could feel emotion about doing this. I used to get excited, but I still feel like a zombie in so many ways and afraid feeling something will trigger AFib.*

Starting around age twelve, I used to dye my hair frequently. I used home kits on my own and when I grew older, through my early twenties, I went to salons to have my hair dyed. I always chose blonde and red shades for my naturally brown hair. The reveal when my hair dried and I saw what my newly dyed hair looked like was one of my favorite feelings. The excitement or disappointment was fun and whatever the outcome, it could always change again. When I started the steps to dye my hair that September night, I hadn't dyed my hair in a long time. I opened the box, put on the plastic gloves, shook the hair dye bottle, squeezed it, and patted the dye into my hair. When I began to wash out the newly set dye in the shower, I felt like I was taking my life back and my personality was returning as well as excitement for the unknown.

I've only been a shell of myself this last month. I do whatever anyone tells me to do, no question. I haven't made any of my own decisions. Dying my hair reclaimed my will to make my own choices and feel excited for small things. As I stepped out of the shower, I wrapped myself in a towel, and wiped the condensation off the mirror to look at my newly tinted blue hair, smiling. *I'm still strong, even if my outside isn't yet.*

Postop with Dr. Washington

About five weeks after surgery, I went in for my checkup with Dr. Washington. His nurse performed a preliminary exam, excited to see I was thriving. Sitting on the exam table, reacting to her positivity, I said, "Doesn't everyone feel this way? So much better?"

She shook her head, "No, you're doing remarkably."

Dr. Washington came in to examine me and was enthusiastic about my progress, too. It was the first time I'd seen him since I'd left the hospital. We sat down at his desk and he grinned widely, something I rarely saw, since he could be very serious.

"You're cleared of all your postsurgical restrictions. You can sit in the front seat as a passenger in a car, resume driving, and—the best news of all for you—no more blood thinner pills. There are no more tests needed to check your levels and you don't have to monitor what you eat. You can even return to work next week if you want to."

"After only six weeks, no way!" I laughed. "I want my promised twelve weeks of time away from work to have fun and be free of stress and responsibility." *My energy's always changing. There are still good and bad days. Rehab starts soon. I don't know how much rest I'll need after the sessions.*

Dr. Washington understood and didn't change my return-to-work date. He told me at the end of the appointment, "You won't see me again in the office for checkups. You can visit anytime or email with questions."

It was bittersweet. Glad I was healthy, we said goodbye. The same day I saw Dr. Cole for another checkup. While listening to my heart with a stethoscope, she took one side out of her ear and said, "I was in the operating room during the surgery to observe the procedure."

This was a surprise to me, as I did not know that had occurred.

"I never saw a heart so relieved to get a rest when they put you on the bypass machine."

Ugh. I guess I was in pretty bad shape. Why didn't I feel worse or feel more symptoms? Maybe I became so used to the symptoms of being unwell I didn't notice them anymore. My body tried to tell me I was sick for so long, but I didn't hear it.

Timeless Existence

During my recovery, I didn't have anything vastly taxing to worry about. Fortunately, I felt so well as I healed that nothing was a major ordeal. If recovery had gone differently and I hadn't felt so well, it would have been much harder. Since checking into the hospital, I had not worn my wristwatch and continued to keep it off at home. Having no plans for days and not having to worry about the time or missing anything was liberating. I enjoyed the freedom that a timeless existence provided. At liberty to do as I wished after a few doctor appointments and my daily walk, I tried to find daytime events that I normally missed while at work and pretended I was a tourist visiting Boston. I went downtown for a Halloween parade and ate lunch at midday food trucks. Some days I preferred to stay at home and catch up on TV shows I was behind on.

In late September, I had a glaucoma appointment scheduled with Dr. Knight. She had recently changed office locations to an office near my condo, and I decided to walk the one-mile distance. The previous day I had walked about ten minutes and my chest hurt; nevertheless, I wanted to try to walk to Dr. Knight's. I progressed slowly, with my chest heaving at times, since there are hills on the way. I made it to the appointment with time to spare; my chest never hurt and I didn't feel the need to take a taxi. During the appointment, I learned to my relief that my eye was stable after the surgery and the transformation I had gone through.

One weekend with my family I went to the L.L.Bean outlet in New Hampshire. I often go to the cavernous store and walk around looking at the merchandise and trying on a large number of clothes. No shopping carts means I have to carry a large, heavy load of clothes into the dressing room. That in combination with extensive walking had always been a challenge for me at this store. On this fall visit, I loaded up my arms with piles of jackets and sweaters. I walked to the dressing room slowly with my heavy pile. *Wow, I can do this. Mom doesn't have to help me carry everything like before during my years with AFib.* On the ride back home, I thought, *I'm not tired. I don't even think I need to rest today and tomorrow like I usually do after these outings.*

The week after the shopping outing, the weather turned hot and humid. Walking caused my chest to hurt and I didn't want to walk a great deal; yet, I persisted since it was doctor's orders. Sitting in my car in the parking lot at a pond, I finished up a call with Mom.

"Emily, I don't think you should walk today. It's very hot out. Go for a walk indoors instead," Mom said on the phone.

"I just got here and I see Sam and Josie waiting for me. I'm going to try," I replied and caught up to Sam and Josie.

"Mom didn't want me to come, but let's see how it goes," I told Sam.

"We can go slow and rest."

On the walk, I kept up with them and did not stop to rest often. Happy to test my limits, I found I could succeed.

Three days later, I received a call from one of the cardiac rehab centers to inform me I could come in for an informational meeting on October 10th. I had to attend rehab at a new hospital where I had never been a patient because MGH couldn't start my sessions until the end of October. *Dr. Cole said there could be a long wait to start rehab, but this is so frustrating! Three months later is too much. Now I'll have to go to work and rehab at the same time. How will I do it?* I tried not to worry about it much because it was a stress I didn't need. Work would be half days at first so I hoped I could manage both if the timing worked out. As I thought about it, I realized I wanted time off to go to New York and I could see Josie while Sam worked. *I'm glad that rehab is starting later. I don't want to give up my commitment-free life yet.*

NYC

I decided to go to New York City for one night in October before starting rehab the following week. I recalled from years of following one of my favorite French cookie brands online that the company's USA headquarters in New York offered a dessert cooking class. The weekly class was held on Wednesdays in Brooklyn. I could not normally attend unless I took time off from work, which I didn't feel was justified. I now had the opportunity to go. I also wanted to test myself to learn how I would do on a short vacation with my new valve. In the past, after my ablations and eye surgeries, I went to New York City on a day trip to test myself in similar ways. These trips helped me regain my self-assurance and discover any snags that might come up while I could easily return home to get to the hospital. After those short vacations, if no obstacles arose, I would feel ready to go on my usual two-week overseas adventures.

On an unseasonably warm day in mid-October, I arrived in New York City. Despite the heat being physically draining, I felt stronger than I had previously. Excited, I looked forward to future vacations where I wouldn't feel as crummy as I had in the past. My parents were in Europe and I didn't tell them I was going to New York. I sent them a picture of me in Times Square to surprise them, and they were flabbergasted to see me standing in front of the building with the New Year's Eve ball on the top.

I decided to go to a hair salon in Brooklyn and get a strip of my hair professionally dyed purple and blue to enhance my dye job from a couple of weeks earlier. It felt like old times being in a salon, and I was pleased with the outcome. During my cooking class, where we made rich chocolate mousse, I had a great time and met fascinating people who worked at fashion houses and large banks in the city. Exploring neighborhoods, sampling foods, and discovering new places during my two-day stay was energizing, and I proved to myself that I could indeed go on a short trip successfully.

I Am Not a Science Experiment

When I returned from New York, I attended my annual doctor appointments. Once when I had an appointment at MGH during college, a technician I had never met read my patient file and said excitedly as she came in to meet me, "Wow, you have a lot of history!"

Thanks, Captain Obvious. Now I'm her prized specimen she gets to examine. This will never end.

During my AFib episodes, I had my period while on blood thinner medication and the blood flow did not stop for several weeks and was extremely heavy. When I reached out to my gynecologist for help, he seemed unsure how to address the issue, indicating that he did not have many patients on blood thinner pills. I gave him the benefit of the doubt and continued in his practice.

In October, I saw my usual gynecologist in what turned out to be my last time as his patient. At this appointment, I dressed in a hospital gown and sat on the exam table. I told my doctor patiently, "I recently had my second open-heart surgery, so I can't fully lie down because my sternum is still broken. It's uncomfortable and feels heavy if I lay completely flat. I need to stay propped up on a pillow throughout the exam."

The nurse in the room set me up with a pillow and I adjusted my gown to point to my leg. "I want to discuss the incisions in my groin area." He quickly looked at them without addressing my concerns and moved his attention upward to my chest.

He pressed down on my chest near my scar and he said, "Wow, look at that!" What he meant was how my chest still caved in and rebounded when he pressed the broken bones. *This doesn't hurt, but it's uncomfortable and I don't think this is medically necessary.*

He pressed on my sternum again for no medical reason as I lay there, staring at the ceiling, silently seething. *My sternum's fine. Dr. Cole would've told me if it wasn't. This is a waste of time.* I did not advocate for myself and tell him to stop and allowed him to continue to play with my body. *He's never seen or touched anything like this before. That's why he's doing it. I feel like a prized specimen again.*

I wish I had said, "Why do you need to press on my ribs?" After I left, I was irate about the experience. I had not felt like an experiment in a long time, and I hated it because it brought back many troubling memories. *I'm not going to be his patient anymore. I won't give him the chance to treat me that way again. I know there's usually only one specialist or surgeon with experience to treat me so I have to tolerate a lot, but not all the time.* This experience helped me to start to find my voice during my recovery and advocate for myself. I had walked in the heat when Mom advised against it—a task I wouldn't have considered in the past. Now, I finally put my foot down and decided I was no longer going to see this doctor.

Denny Makes Feelings Clear

Growing up, I couldn't explain or communicate all of my anger and feelings surrounding my health history. In 2006, when I saw *Grey's Anatomy* on television I finally heard an articulation of how I felt. In the episode "Losing My Religion," a character on the show, Denny, had a heart condition as well. When trying to explain his feelings to his girlfriend he said, "For five years, I've had to live by the choices of my doctors. The guys that cut me open decided my life. There wasn't one choice that was mine."[7]

This is incredible. This is exactly how I feel and didn't have words to say. I called Mabel right away after the show to discuss Denny's statement. She was as excited as I was to see our internal experience reflected.

"Our doctors and bodies have controlled us and made all of our major decisions for us. At times, there is nothing we can do to alter what happens to us," she said.

I agreed. "My body has failed at times when I wanted to do things to live a fulfilling life."

My doctors do not know if I can have children safely, so it's never been something I've pushed for. It feels like another life choice taken away from me before I even had time to think about whether I wanted it or not. Maybe if I was more curious and assertive, I could obtain more direct answers. Growing up without peers to look to as an example, there is only so much I can stand up for. When I want to travel to a new destination with potential risks, I always advocate for myself. Confronting risk-averse doctors and my family is difficult, as I fear disturbing the peace. Other times I worry that pushing for excessive explanations will reveal alarming details that indicate my body is more fragile than I realize.

After my surgery in 2017, while at home recuperating, the same *Grey's Anatomy* episode repeated on television. But this time, my ears rang listening to the latter part of his monologue, "And now I have this heart that beats and works. I get to be like everybody else. I get to make my own decisions, have my own life, do whatever the damn hell I choose."[8]

I forgot he said that. I'm even more like Denny. I too had a heart beating and working better than it ever had previously. Endeavors that had been difficult for so many years gradually became easier. *This is a turning point. Now there are exciting possibilities.* I had never experienced a life where small routine daily tasks were not an ordeal. *My heart might actually have improved since the surgery. Maybe it's not temporary, and things might be better for a long time.*

I, **Emily**, have chosen to devote my time and energy to making my physical and mental health a priority

Target Workload: **4+** M
(METs)

Exercise Card 2.3
Gradually increase / decrease your settings
until reaching your desired workload or intensity (RPE)

Accumulate 45-50 mins. of aerobic exercise
Work towards 10 min. bouts of continuous work
Max. of 25 mins. on each piece of equipment
(unless otherwise approved by Staff)

☐ Treadmill: **20** mins **3** mph **5** %

☐ BioStep: _____ mins   Res. Lvl. _____

☐ Bike 1 or 2.: _____ mins   Res. Lvl. _____

☐ Arm Ergo: **10** mins   Res. Lvl. **3.2**

☐ Elliptical **10** mins   Res. Lvl. **10**

Congrats!

☐ Resistance Training ___ ___ Reps: 8-12 +

Bicep Curls **4** lbs.

Tricep Ext. **4** lbs.

Upright Row _____ lbs.

Shoulder Raises (front) **4** lbs

Shoulder Raise (lateral/side) **4** lbs

Shoulder Raise (overhead) **4** lbs

Sit-to-Stand (squats) _____ sets _____ reps

RPE Scale

| 2 | 3 | 4 | 5 | 6 | 7 | 8 | 9 | 10 |

Last Rehab Session Card (December 2017)

Cardiac Rehab

At the end of October, two and half months after surgery, I began attending cardiac rehab at Mount Auburn Hospital in Cambridge, Massachusetts. As I had never been to this hospital before, I was unsure what to expect. I found it to be a low-key environment with much less chaos than what I was used to at MGH. Although people had appointments and tasks to complete, no one was in a rush, and the atmosphere was much more leisurely.

At first, I had a relaxed attitude toward the rehab sessions, feeling like there was nothing at stake. Dr. Cole had given me the option to stop going if I didn't enjoy it, so I didn't feel fully committed to the experience. I was free to participate as intensely as I wanted, without fear of judgment from anyone. All I needed to do was make sure I could exercise without difficulty, and I was already pretty confident in my ability after my daily walks.

The cardiac department was located at the front entrance of the building. I didn't see much of the hospital because I went straight into the medical suite. This made it feel like my own private world. I walked past the waiting room and let myself into the cardiac department. As I walked down the long white hall to reach the rehab room, I noticed exam rooms with open doors on both sides, where nurses called patients to discuss blood thinner dosages and the familiar whooshing sounds of echoes could be heard. Trying to ignore all the reminders of what I had gone through, I chose to stay focused on what I was there to do and blocked out the noise.

The rehab room contained treadmills, an elliptical machine, exercise bicycles, a weight area, and other exercise machines. At each hour-long session, about five to six patients attended, and a conference room in the corner was used for classes with a dietitian and other specialists. One lead registered nurse and two exercise physiologists set the program for each patient based on their abilities.

Most visits, I had a good time at rehab and looked forward to going. The sessions followed more or less the same pattern every time. I arrived for my session in my workout clothes. A basket at the entrance contained heart monitors. In the same basket was a task card personalized for each patient. We picked these up at the beginning of class as they outlined our exercise routine for the day. We attached cardiac monitors to ourselves. The exercise physiologists kept track of everyone's heartbeats on the EKG monitor overlooking the room, ensuring that we exercised safely. They were looking out for irregular beats or hearing one of us complain about chest pain or shortness of breath, which might indicate our bodies were not ready for exercise.

I attended sessions three times a week with an older crowd. Patients seemed shocked that someone my age would be attending an activity assumed to be only for older people. While putting my bag into a locker at the start of the session, every few days a new patient sidled up to me and asked, "What are you doing here, young lady?"

The first time I was asked this, I opened my mouth and closed it again. *I need a new answer. My old one no longer works.* I paused as the person looked me over to try to find any visual signs of a problem. Tentatively I answered, "I had my second open-heart surgery in August and I got a new valve."

Dumbfounded, her mouth dropped open. She stared at me. "You're so young to have a heart problem. Are you okay now? There's no one else in here who had open-heart surgery."

I nodded and sighed at the response I was used to. *I finally had a common procedure but I'm still the odd one out.* Most people came to rehab for less invasive procedures like stents. *I want to talk about my experience with someone. I'll try to make friends.* While exercising with our heart monitors we listened to music over the speakers in the room. Sometimes patients chose what station we wanted and I preferred pop music rather than classical or jazz, the majority vote. My rehab routine included weightlifting, walking on the treadmill, and using the elliptical. I cycled my arms on the arm ergometer and pedaled my legs on the BioStep. The tasks were personalized based on my abilities, while also pushing me to test and discover new limitations.

I kept a watchful eye on the EKG monitor, searching for any AFib that I couldn't feel, but I never observed any irregularities. Comparing my EKG waves to those of the other patients, even though I didn't really know what I was seeing, was a good way to pass the time. Every EKG wave is like a fingerprint. Everyone has a unique pattern making it interesting to watch the monitor from more of an artistic point of view than a medical one.

Guest speakers visited and, on one occasion, a dietitian taught us healthy eating habits. Although I already followed many of her suggestions, such as reducing sodium and consuming more fish, I found it beneficial to hear her ideas. This talk motivated me to continue eating healthier meals, a habit I picked up during my recovery.

As time went on, I began to realize I could do more than what was asked of me on my task card. At the end of October, eleven weeks postop, I bravely asked one of the exercise physiologists, "Can I please try running instead of walking on the treadmill?"

She thought for a moment and said, "Yes, but you have to wait until I'm standing next to you and watching every step and the monitor. We'll do it at the end of class in case there's a problem and you need to go to the ER."

It sounded daunting but I sensed I would be fine and agreed to her conditions. As the hour-long class ended and patients started leaving the room, I walked over to the machine. I started with walking and gradually increased to running slowly. The exercise physiologist and I monitored my heart rate on the EKG monitor, but nothing unusual was detected. I ran for a couple of seconds, feeling short of breath quickly, but I wasn't exhausted. It was the first time I ran since my surgery discharge on the hospital floor in August and playing with Blueberry and Maxi in September. It felt like a promising start to doing more.

After beginning rehab, I also returned to BollyX, a dance-fitness class. For about a year before the surgery, I had been taking the Bollywood-music-inspired dance aerobics class two times a week and loved it. I am not the best dancer and I'm not very coordinated, so I modified the moves in accordance with my ability and stamina. Sometimes I did less than my classmates, but I always had a great time and smiled throughout the entire class, having fun. Upon my return to class, I noticed an immediate difference. *I don't have to modify what I'm doing. Now I can keep up!* I could fully partake in the activity, jumping and twirling along with everyone else to the upbeat music.

Return to Work and an Epic Walk

I focused on the positives happening for me and my body and tried to stay stress-free when I returned to work part-time on November 6th—ironically, the day my surgery had originally been scheduled. Dr. Washington decided I should slowly ease back into work, working four hours per day. *I like talking with my friends, but I miss my timeless existence.* I continued to attend rehab three days a week.

Ahead of Thanksgiving, I asked the rehab staff if I could try running on the treadmill for longer periods of time. Given the green light, I realized running feels different than before the surgery. *The voice in my head that screams at me to stop is gone. I've reached my limit. I don't have to quit, but I have to rest.* As I grew stronger at rehab, it was rare to hear that voice. I wanted to keep trying new physical activities because I suspected I was capable of doing more than I ever had in my life. On Wednesday, the day before Thanksgiving, I decided to try taking a walk I had never attempted. Daring myself, I wanted to walk from Sam's house to my parents', a six-mile journey. After picking up Josie from Sam's house after work, I walked with Josie while I carried my duffle bag over my shoulder. Before my surgery, I never would have considered walking such a long distance, or even taking a short walk while carrying anything. If needed, I had precautions set in place. If we couldn't continue, Josie and I could always ride the bus running alongside our walking route, or we could wait for Sam to pick us up in her car after she finished work.

We walked at a leisurely pace, and Josie stopped repeatedly and tried to return home since she hates busy roads. I coaxed her along for a while, and eventually, she realized we weren't turning around. As we transitioned from the city to the suburbs, the street grew quieter and we made more progress. I'm not sure exactly how much time the six-mile walk took us, but we spent well over an hour, maybe two, enjoying our time together and taking frequent breaks for Josie to sniff the bakery entrances and trees.

Sam planned to pick us up along the way when she left her office. I texted her updates along the route, letting her know both of us were all right. When we were nearing the final mile, Sam texted to offer to pick us up in her car. I declined, telling her that we would meet her one street away from my parents' house.

She called me after reading my message. "I can't believe you've made it so far already," she said excitedly. "I was sure you'd need me to pick you up. This walk's like a race, and you're approaching the finish line."

I had never run in a race, so I didn't know what that was like, but I felt a sense of achievement. "We're almost there, you better hurry or we'll beat you home!"

Sam never walked the route herself, even though she considered trying it and began sniffling on the phone, "I'm proud you have accomplished such a feat."

Her blue car pulled up alongside us; she had the window down and was smiling with tears in her eyes. "Congratulations!" she shouted out the window.

I laughed and Josie and I happily got into the car after the long adventure. We parked in my parents' driveway and went upstairs. My parents greeted us in the foyer. I put my bag down and said, "Guess what Josie and I just did?"

"Finished working for a few days?" Dad asked.

"NO! Josie and I walked six miles!"

My parents stared at me in awe that I could accomplish such a long walk, especially while carrying my duffle bag. We celebrated the holiday feeling like our burdens were lifted.

Following the Thanksgiving break, I returned to work full-time and continued to attend rehab early in the morning before heading to the office. Carrying on doing the routine exercises on my task card, I started running more. I ran for a couple of minutes and walked at varying speeds and inclines on the treadmill. Continuing to progress, I increased the time I could run at every session. I also bumped up my elliptical level to a higher setting, without anyone requesting I do so. *Rehab will be over at the end of the year. I have to get the most out of it that I can. I need to feel that I've tried my best here.* I had less difficulty exercising, and pushed myself to do more, something I had never been able to do in the past.

NYC Exercise Class

Mabel and I decided it was time for me to visit her in New York for a weekend in the early winter. We went downtown to shop for new glasses for her, and the following day we attended an exercise class together. It was fun to see what each of us could do after a lifetime of limitations and exclusions in a room full of people who had no idea about our conditions. Mabel took on inclines and stairs faster than I could, and she lifted heavier weights than me. Many other people around us surpassed us in speed and difficulty level. *They're so fast, but stay focused on your goals.* I checked out what Mabel could do for curiosity's sake, not competition.

"What do you want to get for dinner?" I panted, not focusing on Mabel's acceleration.

"Let's get sushi," she answered. "You're doing so well on the rower! I bet you can notch it up a level." Thinking about eating more at dinner and Mabel's encouraging words, I tried a little harder.

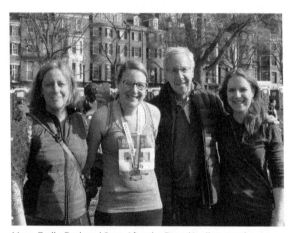

Mom, Emily, Dad, and Sam, After the Race (April 14, 2018)

Becoming an Athlete

Realizing that my body had been transformed and that it wasn't a fleeting occurrence, I set a challenge for myself. I had always thought I might like to walk in the Boston Marathon, sponsored by the Boston Athletic Association (B.A.A.). It would take me approximately twenty hours to walk the 26.2-mile course (not counting bathroom or meal breaks) and it would be exhausting. I didn't see it as a realistic possibility; although I thought about it, I never told anyone. Instead, with my new abilities, I decided to attempt to run in the B.A.A. 5K race, which took place the same weekend as the marathon. The race route covers a 3.1-mile course in downtown Boston, starting and ending in the Common.

I mentioned this idea to the staff toward the end of my time at cardiac rehab. They agreed that it was a good goal to pursue. With the race in April, it would be perfect timing to start training, since I needed something to keep me active and motivated after rehab ended in December. Not knowing the entry requirements, I wasn't sure if I could enter the race. I didn't know if I'd have to qualify with a fast race time or any other prerequisites, but I forged ahead with training because signup was not until January. I didn't want to tell friends or family, since I didn't want to get our hopes up.

In early November, I told Mom about the race because she basically figured out herself that I wanted to do it. She kept it confidential until December when I surprised Sam and Dad by sharing my intention to sign up for the race. They were excited and supportive upon hearing my news. The experience was even more exhilarating as Sam and I had grown up watching the Boston Marathon, and Mom had also volunteered for it.

Mom said, "Even if people say you can't participate in the race, know that I'm so thrilled that you're feeling so strong that you feel it's possible!"

"I don't know if I can really do it. It might be too hard," I responded. *I usually have to quit. I can try, and if needed, I can walk.*

At rehab in early December, I ran one minute and thirty seconds without stopping. My stamina and abilities categorically started to improve. Mom asked me, "Have you told your doctors about the race? Shouldn't you get clearance to participate?" She was being cautious, as she always was. Choosing to be more independent, I made the decision not to ask my doctors in advance. I could see from the monitor at rehab my heart was good, and I was aware when I reached my limit and needed to stop to rest. In mid-December I had a checkup with Dr. Cole and my first echo after the surgery. Dr. Cole said my echo results were great and she was pleased with my progress. I told her—but didn't ask—about the race. She was supportive and never had any doubts about my participation.

My best day at rehab to date was in December when I ran for seven minutes and thirty seconds on the treadmill during the twenty-minute workout. It was an electrifying milestone and I wasn't sure I could repeat it. To my surprise, I continued to advance. This indicated to me I was becoming stronger than ever. Right before Christmas, I ran continuously for two and a half minutes without stopping, twice in eleven minutes.

Once, during high school, Benny escaped from my parents' yard and ran up the street. Sam, Dad, and I all chased after him by running down the center of the road. Because of my concern, I ran faster than Sam and Dad to try to reach Benny as quickly as possible. It was the one time prior to the surgery I had an opportunity to test if I could run faster than Dad or Sam. Previously, I could always run fast, but for only a short period of time, and I burned out quickly, never pushing myself to keep going. I could never run at an even pace over a long distance. At rehab I discovered that I could run at a slower pace for multiple minutes at a time.

Run Club

Cardiac rehab came to an end in December 2017 after I had completed thirty-three sessions. At the same time, I started my own training regimen by downloading a 5K app on my phone that coached me on alternating periods of walking and running with longer increments in each session. To monitor my progress, I purchased a fitness watch.

In January, I signed up for the 2018 B.A.A. 5K race. There were no hurdles or any athletic achievements required for entry. I projected my race finish time to be one hour, which is the maximum time allowed for participants to complete the course and be counted as official finishers. Even if I walked, I could finish the race within the time limit. The race was scheduled for April 14, 2018.

When I told Mabel about my race, she said, "I've learned to not get mad at what my body can't do and be thankful for what it can do. Sounds cheesy but I think it's a good mentality to have. Start where you can and grow what you can." She also promised to come cheer me on, on race day.

As an additional exercise motivator, in mid-January I joined the Adidas Run Base Run Club. This club met twice a week for runs around downtown Boston, and it welcomed runners of all abilities and ages. It was managed out of a store located on the same street as the Boston Marathon finish line, and I started attending one night a week.

All the club members were extraordinarily kind and supportive. Although everyone was training for different races, from marathons around the world to the same 5K as me, we were a team. At ease with the members, I shared my cardiac history with most of them. They were glad that I was trying a new sport and never discouraged me from participating. During our group runs, everyone cheered me on and clapped, regardless of how slowly I ran.

At run club, we ran laps around a track, practiced running up hills in Boston Common, and ran long runs along the Charles River past the Museum of Science. One or two other people slowed their pace in order to run with me as I always found myself at the back of the pack. Even while walking during the runs, I made progress each week. I felt more and more like Benjamin Button as I was able to do so many new things as the weeks advanced. I bought a pair of running shoes from an official sports store to better prepare myself and congratulate myself on my growth.

Mom started calling me Benjamin in emails when I told her about my week's achievements. "Benjamin's a beast!" she'd say, and my confidence grew.

My best day of 5K training was at the end of January. I ran and walked for thirty minutes along the Charles River in Cambridge, used the elliptical machine in the gym for forty-five minutes, and attended a one-hour BollyX dance class, all consecutively. I didn't make progress every time I exercised, though. The day after such a good day, I had a bad one when the group at run club went on a five-mile loop run and I could only make it 0.76 miles. I didn't feel soreness, pain, or heart palpitations, but instead heard the familiar voice in my head telling me to stop because my body had no more to give and I had to quit. It was the first time I felt defeated since joining the club. *A little something is always better than nothing.*

The Word Is Out

In late January I told the rest of my family, friends, and doctors about the race. My athletic accomplishments have never been solely mine, as I have always had doctors and nurses helping me achieve my goals and get to the point where I can participate. The support from family, friends, and doctors during my training was overwhelming, with everyone cheering me on from afar.

All of the positivity helped my self-confidence grow. *Don't be so discouraged at the back of the pack at run club. You don't have to quit or sit it out anymore! Walk if you need to. Set reasonable goals.*

The Race Countdown and Japan Redux

Every step of the way, my family and I celebrated the excitement of the upcoming race. When my race bib with my official number arrived in the mail, I brought it to my parents' house so we could see it for the first time together. Sam and Mom prepared their cameras as I stood in the family room, taking the large white envelope into my hands. I slowly opened it, being careful not to tear anything. Inside was a one-page flyer with the course map and directions for getting to the park, as well as my racer's bib. The bib was a shiny white square with my name in large letters and a black participant number with a tracker on the back. I held it up gleefully for photos.

I made sure to forward every race countdown email I received from the B.A.A. to my family so we could all stay updated. Each week at run club, I took note of the official countdown clock in the window of a store, ticking down the days until race day. *I'm so nervous!* I'd email pictures of the clock to my family with worried emojis every week.

Attending run club consistently helped me make progress. Using my 5K training app to train on my own was also helping me see improvements in my ability. In early March, unconvinced I could reach the app's training goal of running twice for eight minutes consecutively within the thirty-minute time block, I tried and succeeded. Dad said, "I'm at a loss for words! This is beyond amazing!"

Mom said, "2018. The year Benjamin takes over Emily's life and brings all new skills into her orbit!"

I responded, "I feel pressure now to keep achieving new and great things all the time."

Mom said, "Next year you'll conquer the world, of course!"

This is a lot to live up to. But I can keep trying to see what I'm capable of accomplishing.

During my solo training sessions, I ran in my neighborhood park. I perfected my playlist of songs that helped boost my energy and would give me a push to make it to the finish line during the race. Taking a cue from the movie *Cool Runnings*, I also visualized the racecourse as I ran, imagining the streets and curves in the road so that I would be fully prepared for what was to come. I also visualized making it to the end and seeing my family waiting for me. When I visualized crossing the finish line and spotting them, I became teary, full of emotions with no idea what it would really be like to see them on race day.

I wanted to have a prize for myself whether I completed the race in April or not. It brought to mind football games where the winning quarterback was asked in the postgame interview what he was going to do next; he'd respond, "Disneyland." Now I could say, "Tokyo" if anyone asked; I had booked a vacation to Japan departing one week after I finished the race. After the two previously canceled trips, I desperately wanted to make it on *this* trip.

Race Eve

Race week arrived and I was filled with a mix of nerves and excitement for the big day. On Thursday night, two days before the race, I met up with a friend from run club to do a practice run through the course. This was extremely helpful, as it allowed me to familiarize myself with the course and mentally prepare for the turns and hills that I would face on race day. Walking and running through the course ahead of time helped me to pace myself properly during the actual race.

On Friday I went to the Runner's Expo at a convention center in Boston where all the athletes participating in the marathon and other weekend races convened. Booths sold running clothes, shoes, and special energy-boosting foods. *I'm not completely out of my element here. I understand some of this stuff and what the food can do. I'm a runner too, like everyone here.*

Friday night I wanted to have a prerace runner's dinner and my family came over to my condo. We ate spaghetti and meatballs so I could fuel up. I love pasta but had not been eating it during training. It made me excited to eat pasta after a long hiatus and to know it would boost my energy the following day. I asked at the table, "Am I ready now?"

Mom reached over under the table and poked my strong leg muscle. With a smile she said, "Yes!"

After dinner, I prepared my clothes for the next morning. I put on my tank top so I could attach and position my runner's bib to my shirt. Taking the bib on and off about ten times with nerves and striving for perfection, I eventually placed it correctly. *Finally, it's ready and I'm as ready as I'll ever be. There's nothing more I can do now except get a good night's sleep.*

Race Day

Race morning I woke up rested but nervous, having no idea what to expect. *I don't think I can run the entire course. I'll eat a banana with peanut butter for breakfast to be full of energy.* While eating, I checked the weather and learned it was fifty degrees, much warmer than forecast. Although fifty degrees doesn't sound warm, training in Boston in the winter means running in twenty- to thirty-degree temperatures. I had not run in spring temperatures for long because New England winters can linger until the first week of April.

The race was the second weekend of April. I adjusted my running clothes. Putting on my purple sports bra, light gray striped tank top, full-length plain black leggings, purple headband, and teal, neon green, and pink running shoes, I was ready to go.

At 6:30 a.m., I took the subway to the Common, the meeting spot for the start of the race. Exiting the station, I saw that all of the roads usually so busy with traffic and pedestrians were closed and race signs were being erected. Feeling butterflies, I walked over to the Common to the giant white race tents. I met my excited and nervous family at 7 a.m. Not wanting to become emotional, I tried hard to keep myself composed but some tears leaked out of my eyes. I officially checked in at the race tent and received my runner's bag with a shirt and snacks inside.

Mabel came from New York to support me and met me at the race tent. She wore a black tank top that said *ImPossible* to cheer me on. She gave me a hug, saying, "I know you can do it!"

My friends from run club and local friends arrived, and we all congregated together with my family, waiting for the designated time to enter the starting gates. We took lots of pictures, and my run-club friends reviewed my outfit with me to make sure I wouldn't overheat. We also reviewed tips like staying close to the corners when running and not exerting myself too much until the end so I'd have the energy to finish the course.

About thirty minutes before the race commenced, it was time for all of the athletes to enter the starting gate area. Prior to going in, as I handed Mom my valuables, my memory flashed back to the hospital admissions waiting room, where I checked in for my surgery, eight months earlier. I had handed Mom my wallet ahead of the surgery and it was the same exchange happening again, but this time for a much happier occasion. Blinking my eyes once, I focused back on the present and went into the gated area.

Full of excitement and nerves, I stood on the street on the course route, on the other side of the orange gates that separated me from my family. I was next to my run-club friends, feeling jittery but also soundly supported. For the first time, I was trying to achieve an athletic goal on my own, rather than watching from the sidelines. Trying not to become overwhelmed, I suddenly heard the starting gun, and the elite runners were off. My race had begun!

The 10,000 participants and I were seeded by predicted run time. By the time my friends and I made our way toward the starting line, fifteen minutes had passed and the elite runners had already completed the race. Eventually, it was my turn to advance to the starting line, away from my family, and I turned and saw them as I went around the corner on Beacon Street. We waved goodbye, and it was time to start my journey. Until I was nearing the finish, I wouldn't see them again. Turning on my music playlist, I ran over the starting line with my friends.

It's GO Time

As planned, my friends peeled off as we crossed the starting line and I was soon on my own. To calm my nerves, I told myself *running today is no different than all the times you went before. It's like Thursday when you practiced the course. Don't run faster, go at your normal pace.* People passed me the entire time, but there were also people walking behind me as I weaved in and out of the crowd.

Time was strange. *I feel like I've run so far, but my watch says I've only gone a short distance.* Other times, I felt that I had barely progressed but then saw the first bright yellow mile marker far sooner than expected. *These weren't here on practice night. I'm really moving.* I texted Sam when I saw one so she'd have an idea where I was on the course.

My music playlist was set up so that I knew which songs should come on during certain miles if I was following my expected pace. *I'm on track.* It was thrilling running by the closed stores and down the center of the busy streets, something a pedestrian could never normally do. My running bib said my name and strangers on the sidelines called out for me, cheering and shouting supportive phrases to keep me going, "You got this ... Almost there ... GO Emily!"

There was a tunnel on the route right before the halfway point, where runners, including me, screamed to make an echo as we passed through it. Afterward, we ran up a small hill as we came back out through the tunnel on the other side. *It's so hot, I won't make it up the hill.* Nevertheless, I made it up slowly and never stopped. Keeping my eyes staring ahead, trying not to notice how much further until the street evened off, helped me progress.

Almost at the top of the next hill, I saw mile marker two. It was a welcome sight after the two hills. *Almost there, one mile to go!* Panting, I turned a corner onto the street where the run-club store was located. Running by the headquarters was invigorating and I kept going, down the street, to the official Boston Marathon finish line. As I ran over the freshly painted street banner with a wide yellow border with blue block letters outlined in white, I took a picture of myself. This was easy to do because I was so slow. Further down the road, I saw the final stretch of the course. *I can make it to my finish line if I keep trying.*

Since so many of the runners were faster than me, most of them were finished by the time I reached the second mile. I was virtually by myself many times throughout the course. As I neared the end, I saw a friend with his wife and Boston terrier puppy watching me from the sidewalk. There were fewer spectators, so I could easily call out to him, wave, and say "hi" as I ran by. They were the first familiar faces I'd seen since leaving the starting line.

Turning off my music, I immersed myself in the moment. I saw Sam, her then boyfriend (now husband), Dad, and Mabel. They screamed and cheered for me, taking photos and videos, running beside me as I neared the end, with about .15 of a mile to go. I smiled back and waved, experiencing a tiny boost of energy. It was good timing since I was weary. The street curved as I passed mile marker three, and I left my cheerleaders; gates that led up to the finish line kept them from following me.

To stop myself from slowing down, I played Sia's song "Alive," which helped me keep pace. *No one's holding me back anymore and I'm still alive. I survived all of the struggles, surgeries, and recoveries throughout my lifetime.*

As I turned left on the course, nearing the end, I saw my friends from run club standing behind the orange gates, screaming and cheering, running beside me with signs. As I approached the finish line, the official race time clock loomed closer. Sam and Dad raced to the street where I was and filmed my finish. My run-club friend had advised me to save some energy for the end of the course because, if I felt up to it, I could try to sprint over the finish line. Ready to do it, I took off fast. Everyone was shocked I ran so fast at the end. I heard Sam and Dad's astonishment in the video they recorded. My family thought I would be exhausted at the end, but I showed them what Benjamin Button could do.

I briefly paused after the finish line, as I leaned down and a volunteer put a yellow-and-blue ribbon with a large silver unicorn medallion (the mascot of the B.A.A.) around my neck. *I'm not full of emotion like I thought I'd be. I'm glad to stop running since I have a stitch in my side now.*

My inner strength and determination paid off. I never walked or stopped to rest for the entire length of the course. In hindsight, I could have run faster, as I was not out of breath at the end.

After I received my medal, Mom wanted more photos, so I continued running a short distance further until I was out of the gates and reunited with everyone. Instead of worrying about my finishing time, I remained focused on the present moment.

I was encircled with lots of hugs from my family and friends. They all fussed over me, offering water and snacks, but I declined as I was just happy to stop running. We walked over to the grass and took pictures with my new finisher's medal. The other members of the run club made their way over to take victory photos with me since I was the last of our group to complete the race.

Being with all of my friends, my family, and the club members was the most special part of the day. I said goodbye to my run-club friends as they returned home and I stayed with my family and friends. As we caught up, we noticed a local news station broadcasting stories about the race. Sam approached them and asked if they wished to interview me, and they agreed.

Spreading the Word about My Accomplishment

I went over to the cameraman and the reporter to learn what to do for my interview. I shared my story with the reporter, and she informed me in advance about what she might ask. Despite being nervous, I didn't mind all the attention and publicity about something I usually kept so private because I was so happy after completing the race.

The live news broadcast began; I stood across from the reporter with a giant smile. She asked me, "Why is it a special day for you?"

Rocking side to side a little with nerves, I said, "It's my first athletic event ever."

"Tell me what you mean and about the trials you have been through."

"I was born with a congenital heart condition and had my first surgery at age six and my last surgery was in August, so this was my first, big sporting event!"

She was shocked and said, "Ever! You never did anything sport-like before?"

I shook my head. "No gym class, nothing."

She asked, "How did the race go for you?"

"Great!"

She said, "You have an incredible story, Emily. Thank you so much for joining us and congratulations on your first ever sporting event and your first 5K! That's really incredible!" She waved her arms around excitedly when she said "ever" and clapped my shoulder as she said congratulations.

We spoke after the cameras turned off and I returned to my family and friends. I was pleased that I put myself out there and shared my story. Later, Mom's friend, who happened to be watching TV at home, texted me to say that she saw me live on the program. By chance, she had turned on the television to that specific station, and there I was.

Post-interview, some of my friends left and the rest of us went out for a celebratory lunch at 11 a.m. I was relieved to sit down for the first time since I had departed from my house for the race that morning. *I'm not tired, but I don't want to stand much longer.* Indulging in a lunch with items I had avoided for months, like dessert and orange juice, was a real treat that I savored.

After lunch, and a great day spent together, Mabel returned to New York. While I was walking with my family through the park after lunch, I had a private moment with Dad. I said proudly to him, "When I was a baby, you didn't think I could do this."

He replied, "You sure showed them!" I had proven to all of the doctors and everyone who might have doubted me throughout the years what I could now do.

Later, I went to Sam's house and wore my medal proudly the entire day, even while walking through the grocery store. The following morning, I woke up at 8:30 feeling pretty good. *I can't wait to see pictures and tell everyone about what I did!* Going through pictures, sending out emails, and posting on Facebook about my accomplishment took up most of the morning. I was notified of my official race finish time, not much less than a walking time. My time wasn't great, since my running abilities never advanced much more beyond what I could do in February. I never became faster, but I remained steady. *At least I didn't stop to walk or to rest along the course.*

My tracking watch has been wrong this entire time! It says I ran 3.4 miles, but the race is only 3.1. The distances I thought I'd practiced running were incorrect. Race day turned out to be the first time I actually ran a 5K distance without stopping and walking. After all of the training and preparation, I was stronger than I even thought I was.

Responses to My Race and Postrace Thoughts

I heard back from doctors, family, and friends after I sent out emails and posted on Facebook about my race. Everyone was proud of my participation. Perhaps the most special response of all came from Dr. Smith. I hadn't seen or spoken with him since I was in the hospital in August. He was always included on my emails about my recovery and progress, but he never responded. After the race he wrote, "Wow—you are and always have been spectacular." Since middle school, he had never been a proponent of exercise, so reading his note made me feel good. I still didn't feel like I accomplished much because I might have been able to do even more but, for now, I was happy everyone else was so happy.

Dad wrote me an email the following day after the race, "Congratulations on finishing! And even running the whole way! It's great you set a very high goal for yourself, worked so hard to reach it, and succeeded with flying colors!"

Having never had a sports goal or another dream in life, it felt good to know I could set my mind to something and complete it. Even my travels were more like small wishes, hoping no medical procedures got in the way and forced me to cancel. Since I was gradually building up to the race, it became my first big goal, and my body didn't stop me from reaching it. People now called me—of all people—an athlete, and I began to believe it, a small bit. Maybe I could successfully have tiny athletic dreams.

Mom said, "My daughter the jock," something I'm not sure she could have ever imagined saying about me.

I spent the weekend taking it easy, not doing anything too active, and was back to my new self on Monday, needing no further recovery. Days later, Dr. Cole sent me an email, "We have an opportunity to highlight some patient experiences on the MGH ACHD [Adult Congenital Heart Disease] website and after I viewed your news video, I thought it might be wonderful to highlight you!"

"Sure." I wrote back. *I hope I can inspire other patients.*

The week after the race went by quickly, and then I traveled to Japan. Finally, after all of my trip cancellations, I made it. I spent a week in Tokyo, which was my favorite city from my previous visit. A lot had changed since 2009. It was no longer uncommon to see foreigners, and many of my favorite things about Tokyo had become rare. Elaborately decorated fingernails, high schoolers dressed in various costumes ranging from punk to baby doll in the Harajuku neighborhood, and some trendy food items were no longer as prevalent.

I chose to visit zoos to keep myself busy when I couldn't repeat some of the experiences. Each day, I took the train several hours outside of Tokyo to do this and had more authentic experiences as I went further and saw fewer foreigners. I loved playing with monkeys and lemurs. I also visited with friends, shadowed them in their daily lives, and ate interesting foods while seeing the sights together. After an eventful two weeks, I came home.

I noticed that I had made a couple of physical improvements following the race. I maintained the weight I had lost with my new diet and exercise regimen, and lifting weights made me stronger. When I went to Japan, lifting my suitcase was noticeably easier than usual. I focused on my accomplishments and considered how I could help my family experience the same success. I inspired Mom to try riding a bike and swimming after an absence of many years. She became "Benjamin 2." I not only tried new physical things, but I was ready to make other changes as well.

David Bowie

In March 2016, I watched a documentary film about David Bowie and was struck by something he said: "You can wake up and still change your life." I carried this thought with me every day as I sat at my office desk, feeling like my life was wasting away. For years, I felt stuck and frustrated, going through my daily routines, not knowing how to transform my situation. Subsequently, a change occurred in March 2018.

Outside forces intervened and I resigned from my job in HR without another job lined up. This caused me to feel sad, angry, and nervous about this sudden change in my life. In a professional development class, I took a quiz about change and I was rated at ninety-nine percent of hating change—not surprising, as my fear of change had kept me at my despised desk for years. I have always found comfort in planning, being prepared, and knowing what lies ahead because so many unforeseeable things have happened to me.

Coincidentally, David Ortiz posted a picture on his Facebook account the week I left my job, holding a sign, "Emily, You Got This." It was for another Emily, who was fighting cancer; nevertheless, I saved the photo and set it as the home screen on my phone because it gave me hope. I tried to see the positive in this negative situation. Leaving my job happened while I was training for the 5K. One night before starting a group run I let a run-club friend know about my change in employment status and she said, "You'll have so much more time to train now."

I laughed, since the thought was at the back of my mind, too, and we valued the same nonwork priorities.

I have never been a career-driven person. Muddling along through the years, surviving, I never figured out what I wanted to do with my life. Career tests have always suggested administrative positions for me, and I stumbled upon my job in HR purely by chance. My top priority has always been my health, which has sometimes limited my career options, as I require good health insurance and pharmacy benefits. I prefer a predictable routine, and working in an office all day puts minimal strain on my body. If I feel unwell, I can sit and I don't have to walk around much. No one relies on me for urgent problems. This also allows me to manage my absences, planned or otherwise, without disrupting work. I have held jobs that offer generous time off for doctor's appointments. My health concerns rarely interfere with my work, so I have not needed to disclose them. My sole career goal has always been to retire, and understanding how people could like spending time at work was a foreign concept to me.

As an adult, opportunities to change everything and reevaluate one's goals and aspirations are rare. Now I had the chance. With the security of having income and health benefits for a few months after leaving my position, less pressure was on me to make a rushed career decision. Grateful to survive everything, I wasn't taking advantage of what life had to offer and wanted to find a new path. *I can seize this opportunity and still change my life, like David Bowie said. But I'm still not strongly interested in anything. I need to start somewhere.* I checked out career books from the library and took tests about job skills but wasn't inspired by anything. *Think outside the box. I'm always saying to myself, my life's wasting away, and I'm not experiencing anything. Don't be negative. When were my happiest times? When did I feel like life wasn't passing me by ... Vacation, at camp, and study abroad.* Camp and study abroad were similar. I lived in a communal setting away from home with people who became my friends. Food was prepared for me and there was a set time when programs ended and I would return home. *When I'm away from home and busy with a group of friends, I'm the happiest.*

What could I do going forward? I'm too old to get a working holiday visa to live abroad. I don't have special skills to qualify for an extended work visa overseas. So what else can I do? I can't live somewhere in the United States that's rural without access to modern medical facilities or specialists. I don't want to be away from my family and friends for an indefinite amount of time. I hadn't lived more than a couple of miles away from MGH since college and I'd always been near my family and friends.

I've always wanted to live and work in Antarctica after that book I read about someone who worked there for a few months. It seemed like a similar environment to camp, with people doing everything together in one place. I was qualified for some job openings in Antarctica and applied. It's a highly competitive place to get a job and people who return from years past get first priority. *I probably can't pass the health exams if I even get an interview.*

One of the career books I checked out from the library proposed taking a seasonal job, which is a short-term job during set times of the year. I knew about seasonal retail jobs but never knew that nonretail seasonal opportunities in a place far from my home base existed. *I don't want to stay near home and I don't want to move around frequently from place to place.* Backpacking and camping are not for me, and I enjoy getting to know an area in depth. *I want constants. I want a job that fits my limits.*

Alaska

Alaska! I had never been to Alaska and didn't know much about it. Growing up, I had a map of Alaska hanging in my parents' dining room, thanks to Grandma who brought it back for us after her trip there. I looked at the map every night during dinner and admired the pictures of animals and adventures throughout the state. Although I never consciously thought about visiting, the images of the animals and adventures were always in my mind. As I searched for new opportunities, I discovered that Alaska had many seasonal jobs available. Among them was an HR position with a nationally known company, which caught my attention. *I can build new skills that will look better on my resume if I decide to stay in HR. The job's in a hotel, not a university, like I've been in for years. It's indoors in an office. I don't have to worry about doing a physical job.* Alaskan cities have hospitals and I could fly home for treatment if needed.

I applied for the job, and less than one week after leaving my university job in March, I accepted an HR position in Denali National Park to start in May. It was impulsive and I was excited. Preoccupied with the race and preparing for Japan, I had little time to research Denali. I blindly accepted the offer. I didn't think too much about my new job duties or what working in Alaska would be like. I viewed it as a vacation with a job during the day, with fewer job responsibilities and a large pay cut. *I can't figure out another career path for now, so why not? I can take an adult sabbatical from May to September and figure stuff out. I don't leave for a couple of months so I can keep reading career books and try to decide what I want to do when I come home.*

Many people saw my decision to change my life and move to Alaska as a brave move. It was scary, but I felt a strong desire for something different. People who knew me well were surprised, as I tend to live within a protective cocoon to shield myself from unpredictable circumstances, so they assumed I was risk averse. While they were right in some ways, I was ready for a temporary change of scenery. Alaska would be a big change, but I was willing to let go of my usual need for control and predictability.

Preparing to Move

Prior to accepting the job, I didn't ask any of my physicians if I could move to Alaska. With my newfound confidence, I informed my doctors of my decision and made it clear that I wasn't seeking their permission, similar to when I told them I was running the 5K instead of asking. Once they accepted my decision, we worked together to prepare for my departure.

Drs. Cole and Knight recommended medical facilities and physicians in Seattle when I asked for referrals to local doctors with expertise in cardiac and ophthalmic care. In order to receive specialist care, I would need to drive from my new Alaskan home to an airport at least two hours away in the city of Fairbanks or four hours away in Anchorage, and then fly to Seattle. That would be a big change from my short drive to MGH.

A health clinic was located a thirty-minute drive away from my new hometown in Denali. I called to learn about their facility. They did not have any capabilities to perform an eye-pressure test, but they did have an EKG machine. I was ready to accept any potential consequence of my isolation because it was more important to me to go to Alaska than worry about the what-ifs.

Time flew by in the spring as I prepared for the race, Japan, and Alaska. Reading career books consumed a lot of my time. Although I did read about some Alaskan tourist activities, my focus was mainly on packing. In April, as I flew to Japan, I watched the tracking map on my airplane-seat TV screen. When we flew over Alaska, I got up from my aisle seat and looked out of the emergency exit door window. I saw nothing but snow and mountains, the white expanse seeming to go on forever. This would be my new home in two weeks, and anticipation filled my stomach with butterflies. I came home from Japan late Friday night and flew to Alaska early Monday morning, commencing one of the greatest adventures of my life.

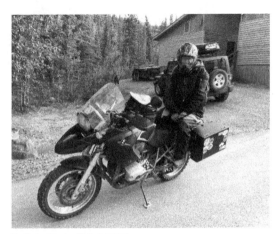

Emily in Alaska (July 5, 2018)

Adventuring in Alaska

In Alaska, "Live your dreams and be free" became my mantra. I arrived in Anchorage during the second week of May, where I was greeted by a cold yet welcoming atmosphere. With one afternoon and evening in the city before departing, I toured the main downtown area. Rows of tourist shops on the streets sold native crafts, furs, gold, and local delicacies such as smoked salmon. There was a mall with outdoor clothing stores and many stands advertising tours around the state. For dinner, I tried a caribou hamburger, which tasted similar to beef, and quickly went to bed, struggling with jet lag from having switched between Japanese, Boston, and Alaskan time zones.

The following day, May 8, 2018, I moved to Denali Park Village in Denali. I would be working in HR at a hotel for tourists visiting Denali National Park, living in a dorm, and eating my meals in the employee dining room. Upon my arrival after a four-hour bus ride, snow was still on the ground up to my ankles in some parts of the village and it was cold out, in the forties. The buildings were constructed of dark brown timber, resembling cabins in the woods, and the property was surrounded by tall spruce trees with the glacial-fed Nenana River bordering it. Employee housing quarters were separate from the hotel, with only a little overlap between walkways.

Less than thirty minutes after arriving at the village, I caught sight of a moose a few feet away. The gigantic brown creature was bending down, busy munching on some grass in a melted patch of snow. The moose was not intimidating since it made no noise and merely glanced at me when I was near. Seeing at least one animal a day was one of the goals I had set for myself before leaving home for Alaska, and I had already seen a moose. As we pulled my suitcase to my room, I remarked to my new boss, "I made the right decision to move here!" My room was located at the end of a long, low building that also housed five other dorm rooms. Each room had a bed, a desk, an area to hang clothes, and a private bathroom. Nothing fancy, very minimal, but I was glad to have heat and a window looking into a wooded area.

On my first day at the village after unpacking, my boss drove me the eight miles from our home to Denali National Park for a short tour. We rode a couple of miles into the park and saw moose, hares, ptarmigans, and caribou. Seeing Mt. Denali was a significant highlight, as only thirty percent of visitors to Alaska get to witness the towering, white, snowy peak owing to poor weather conditions and cloud cover. I was fortunate enough to see it on my first day, however, which was an auspicious start to my time in Denali.

I settled into my new life and job. I began working in the HR office, where I assisted with onboarding the revolving door of new employees, submitting employment verification documents, shuffling housing arrangements, and handling interpersonal conflicts among coworkers. Many times, in my department of two, I was the lone person working. I learned how to help employees from around the world with different backgrounds who spoke little English or had never previously held a job.

I quickly made friends with people who worked in all the departments around the hotel, from housekeeping to food services, from actors to bus drivers. Living and working together made it effortless to spend time with one another. Our work schedules varied, which meant our time off didn't always overlap, but I had made enough friends that I always had someone to talk to in the dining hall or while walking around the village. I fit into our community well even though I was many years older than most of the other 250 employees, who were in their early twenties.

With a lot to do every day at the village after work, the most popular activity was going on hikes. My friends and I went on many hikes in the woods surrounding the village. They were experienced outdoor enthusiasts. *Don't feel intimidated. A hike is a walk.* Usually, I was behind everyone on the hike and pushed myself to keep up. I couldn't always do it, but my friends quickly learned that I was slower than them. They were patient enough to slow down or call out directions if they went too far ahead for me to see the direction they had gone on the trail. I never explained why I wasn't as fit as they were, and they accepted me for who I was.

Every day after work at five, I went for a walk alone before dinner. I walked along the wide shoulder of the highway that was the single road outside where I lived. I saw the river flowing, looked into forests at spruce and birch trees, and often ventured off of the path to explore more. Once, during a solo walk after work, I wandered around looking at lichen and colossal melting ice chunks flowing down the river near the village and got lost in the woods because the trails were not marked. *I'm lost, but I can still hear the highway nearby.* I kept listening for cars and continued to head in their direction. *The midnight sun's still shining and I'll find my way back to the street. I have my bear spray. I've made it through other tough times, I will get out of this too.* I found my way out an hour later, a short distance away from the village. My phone service didn't work in Alaska, so I relied on myself, and grew in confidence after every experience. *I knew I could do it!*

Don't Waste an Alaskan Second

As seasonal employees, my friends and I could partake in tourist activities for a discount. I tried to live up to my London semester abroad motto of "Don't waste a second" and participated in as much as I could. Taking advantage of every opportunity coming my way, I went rafting down a river with rapids, choosing after a few too many high waves to float in the water behind the raft, hanging on by a rope instead of staying in the boat, which was too scary for me. My friend and I flew in a small plane around Mt. Denali, which was the scariest thing I did because I hate turbulence, and we landed on a glacier. The second week in May, I visited five-week-old Alaskan Husky sled-dog puppies and took an all-terrain vehicle (ATV) tour with a couple from Germany and a tour guide. It was freezing cold, and the four-person ATV was open like a golf cart. The company lent me a warm suit to wear over my winter coat, and an employee put a fleece blanket over my legs to keep me warm on the journey. The experienced seven-husky-dog team pulled the ATV through the woods instead of the ATV motor powering us through the forest and around the property. We went through dirt trails, streams, and deep mud puddles, splashing mud everywhere. The dogs loved it and barked impatiently when we stopped because they wanted to keep running. It reminded me of the dog-sled ride I went on in Norway many years before. Although it was chilly, it was an entertaining and thrilling thing to do, requiring little exertion on my part.

During my time off in Alaska, I traveled around the state to participate in many adventures. I drove a motorized ATV, went on a six-wheel-drive army truck tour of the Stampede Trail (of *Into the Wild* fame), and rode the official tour buses into Denali National Park several times to see wildlife. I also saw the aurora borealis and went swimming in freezing lake water on July 4th. On a crab-fishing boat, I saw enormous crabs, and I held one that was the width of my shoulders across and from about my chest to my belly button vertically. Missing the classic salmon run, I did see a couple of shiny silver salmon with big jaws and sharp white teeth swimming upstream.

Walking halfway across a long suspension bridge near Denali was terrifying, and I was too scared to make it all the way across. With nothing but a ravine below me and strong winds shaking me and the bridge, I chickened out and returned to the start. In August, I attended the state fair, where I saw small pigs racing each other, squealing with delight, and lumberjack shows with burly men chopping wood as fast as they could. In the evening I went to a show where I saw monster trucks roaring across dirt mounds, shooting fire bursts from their cabs. I also rode the Alaska Railroad train on several adventures, sat in the glass-top carriage, and ate huge meals of spaghetti and reindeer sausage.

During the summer I attended the World Eskimo Olympics and saw sport competitions in several fields: the Two Foot High Kick; the Knuckle Hop, where athletes see how far they can go in a push-up position with their elbows bent and knuckles down, only toes and knuckles touching the floor as they hop across, to display strength and pain endurance; and the Ear Weight Contest, where competitors hang sixteen-pound weights from their ears and walk along a designated route until the weight drops, in order to demonstrate the ability to withstand frostbite pain.

In September, I saw the annual moose rut, when the humongous males locked horns to battle over females in the park. On a day trip to Fairbanks, I went gold panning and found an ounce or two, which was put into a necklace. I also watched bald eagles eat fish at close range with their sharp yellow talons scooping up their prey from the water below.

At the village I frequently attended the nightly dinner-theater show and became friends with the actors. I took part in other theater activities and enjoyed watching the local singers, many of whom were my talented coworkers. For Halloween, we celebrated Denaliween, and I wore a fake mustache sticker to a party and enjoyed free candy. We celebrated the winter holidays on August

25th (as most National Parks staff do), and I participated in a gift swap with the actors. I created and hosted a Paint-Your-Own Antler Night for the employees at the village, so we'd have a local caribou keepsake when we returned home.

Every day I logged in my journal the animals I saw and the number of each species. I saw black and brown bears with their cubs, and hares whose coats changed from winter white to summer brown. No animal ever scared me, and I wanted to take many home with me. I also went on two whale-watching tours, where I witnessed the spectacle of calving glaciers—one of my favorite sights in Alaska. Massive ice chunks split from the large glaciers and crashed into the water below. I took a glacier canoe tour and hiked on the surface of a glacier. *It's like the glacier in Iceland, but I don't feel crummy hiking like I did back then.* If there was an opportunity to see an animal, go on a tour, or experience something new, I grabbed it.

Maintenance Work

Sitting in my office every day, I was sedentary and bored. When I walked to lunch, I saw my friends from maintenance working in new locations on new projects. Intrigued, I inquired about interning in their department, as I am interested in home repair and enjoy working with my hands. The maintenance department had a full staff of experienced employees in different maintenance fields, making it an ideal place for me to learn. Luckily, my HR manager permitted me to work in the maintenance department a couple of days a month, and I seized this opportunity to learn new skills.

Having a job outside of the usual office environment was quite a different experience for me. I enjoyed being outdoors, even on the days when it was hot, cold, or rainy. It was liberating being in an open space with many different goings-on instead of the usual office machines and predictable customers. Calls came over the radio and we never knew what was next. We assisted guests with varying concerns, from adjusting the heat in their rooms to removing wasp nests on their porches.

I experienced many firsts during my days working in this department. On my first day on the job, I helped take apart an exhaust fan on the roof of the employee dining room building. If I hadn't taken this job, I would never have seen the hotel property from this point of view. As I worked, I waved to my friends below as they passed by and saw me high above the trees. Taking nails out of a board, using an electric screwdriver, and trying to do some wire stripping were not jobs I was good at, but I enjoyed being on the roof. That same day, I worked in the boiler room for one of the hotel guestroom buildings, where I put glycol into a machine to heat the water and learned how the process worked. I'd never even heard of glycol and found out it was a type of antifreeze. In the employee dining room kitchen, I worked on the industrial dishwasher. After power washing the inside of some tubing, I used a pick to remove all of the gray gunk clogging the pipe. This turned out to be my favorite job of the day. Later, I went into a guest room, where I lay on my back underneath a sink vanity, wearing a headlamp to unscrew a faucet pipe. Working in HR, I rarely saw inside the hotel guest rooms and did not interact with guests, so this gave me the opportunity to meet new people and learn more about the property I represented.

At the end of my first maintenance day, I was happy with all that I did and everything I learned. At dinner that night, my friend asked as she routinely did each day, "How are you?"

Instead of my usual response of "OK," without even thinking, I replied, "Good." *I never say that when I'm asked how I am. I must be on the right track.*

Three days later, I returned to work in maintenance and used the chop saw in the workroom to make a doorstop for a hotel room. The noisy saw and shiny silver blade were scary, and sawing was not a task I enjoyed since I was afraid of losing my fingers. Back in the boiler room, I worked on a pipe leaking glycol and used a special sticky material to clog the hole to try to keep the pipe from leaking. It didn't work, and my colleague and I attempted to use some strong tape, but that also proved unsuccessful. Normally, at the office jobs I've had in the past it's not acceptable to fail and work has to be accurate. I was learning that in maintenance work, it was okay to fail and keep trying. It was perfectly all right if everything wasn't perfect the first or second time around.

My best day in the maintenance department was the day I got to drive a yellow-and-black CAT Lift Truck. It reminded me of the Legos bulldozer toy. Something similar to a joystick inside the cab of the truck controlled the direction I drove. My colleague directed me to pretend I was playing a video game in order to use the joystick correctly. Even though I hadn't played a video game in a long time, I remained calm and figured it out. After practice driving in circles around an abandoned lot, I picked up large wooden pallets using the front forks on the truck and transported them elevated in the air to trash piles around the village where I deposited them. I felt proud of myself for not crashing into anything or dropping any of the pallets. Everyone at the village was surprised when they looked inside the truck and saw me driving.

Toward the end of my stay in Alaska, my maintenance colleagues and I began to winterize the village by performing seasonal shutdown procedures. The hotel closed in September for the season, after all the staff left, remaining untouched until it reopened the following April for maintenance workers to set everything up for the upcoming season. In addition to signage, there was a gold mining re-creation with a long trough coming out of a windmill, all of which couldn't be brought inside for the winter. We wrapped everything in plastic to protect it from the soon-to-arrive snow.

Typical shutdown tasks involved going into guest rooms after the last guests had departed to remove the shower heads, turn off the water supplying the toilets, and drain the toilet tanks to prevent the water from freezing over the cold winter and bursting the pipes. We also blew out the excess air and water in the pipes running under the buildings. This meant holding tightly onto hoses as water and air came shooting out at extremely high pressure. Shutdown days were tiring and I found it difficult to keep up with my colleagues, often needing to rest. *I've reached my limit and I can't continue shutdown work. I did so much, I can't dwell on this.*

The team decided to assign me to a different job. I worked in the wastewater department on my final day as a maintenance worker. Many people think waste-water treatment is an unclean job, but in a way, it turned out to be a fun, clean place to work. I climbed up and down tall metal stairs to reach the catwalks. Vacuuming waste from colossal water tanks and using a large spray hose to clean the inside of a tank was amusing. *Don't think about what you're fishing for or cleaning up. Nothing smells bad, it only smells like chlorine.* With so many cleaning procedures to perform on myself and the equipment I didn't worry about the germs I was near. *This is so much easier than shutdown work and I'm still being helpful.* At the end of my five days working in maintenance over the summer, I thought, *I'm glad I stepped out of my comfort zone of daily office work. Working beyond the confines of a cubicle and doing physical tasks is fun. People are more flexible and give me a chance to try things. I should think about this for future career ideas.*

Cool Rider

One of the most exciting things I tried for the first time in Alaska was riding on a motorcycle with a friend. I decided to do this in Denali, where the highways were less crowded and the risks seemed lower than riding on the busy and hectic streets of Boston. My friend drove me all around the park and even on the highway, which was a thrilling experience. After my first ride, I was eager to go again.

When we rode together, I held onto the metal handle bars on the side of the bike, alongside my hips, and I gripped onto the bike with my thighs and calves. I preferred holding the side bars rather than holding onto my friend as it was more comfortable for me. On my second ride with him, he asked me, "Would it be okay with you if I accelerate quickly as we leave the rest stop and merge back onto the highway?"

I thought for a second and had no concerns. It sounded exciting. "Of course." Suddenly, we accelerated and the gravitational force and wind pushed my torso backward. I tried to grab onto my friend as I fell backward and shouted out to him, but he couldn't hear me because of our helmets. Nothing I could do kept me from falling backward. I couldn't stay in the seated position I had been in moments earlier, but my legs were still astride the motorcycle. Lying flat on my back, I gripped the side handle bars, and clenched my thighs tightly against the bike and waited for my friend to notice as we zoomed along.

I wasn't scared as I was parallel to the ground, looking up at the sky. *I'm going to survive. This is not a scary thing like getting chest tubes out. Even if I die or have an accident, I won't regret it. I'm finally really living! He'll figure out that I've disappeared. Once he slows down, I can sit up again.* To enhance my excitement as we zipped along, I sang the lyrics to "Wild and Free," feeling I was living my dreams, having never experienced something so exhilarating.

After about ten seconds, my friend saw I wasn't in his rearview mirror and he quickly slowed down and pulled over, frightened. "What happened?! I'm so sorry. Are you okay? Are you upset?"

I sat up as the forces and wind subsided. *I'm glad I didn't have an accident and something so risky turned out OK.* My heart never sped up with fear and I was fine. "When I agreed to go for a ride, I understood the risks," I told my friend. "I'm not upset. It was great."

"That's a good mentality to have when riding a motorcycle," he replied, relieved.

When we returned to the village, I told my friends about what had happened. A friend with years of riding experience said grimly in his Texas accent, "You would have broken all of your ribs and probably most of your other bones if you fell off the motorcycle." *Eeks, well I'm not upset. I survived everything so I could have such an amazing experience.*

My New Year Begins

While I was in Alaska, I celebrated my birthday in July. For the first time as an adult, I didn't mind that it was my birthday. I usually become discouraged because I feel every year has been the same as the last and I haven't done anything special. That year, I finally got everything out of life I could. Mom emailed me an encouraging message: "I can't wait to see what Benjamin gets up to this year! You have totally embraced your new world; seen that all sorts of new things are possible with a new mindset and more physical prowess." Dad said I looked younger than a year ago because of all my healthy endeavors. I didn't know what adventures would come in my next year, but I looked forward to them. I felt strong going into my last few months living in Alaska.

One Year Surgeryversary

In August, around the time of my one-year surgery anniversary ("surgeryversary"), I felt excited to celebrate the good year I had experienced. Prior to celebrating, though, I had to get through some tough times. In the weeks leading up to the August date, I experienced many memories and flashbacks of what I went through one year before. As I remembered the upsetting tests at the hospital and my feelings in the weeks leading up to the surgery, some stress and sadness returned.

I had some irregular heartbeat flutters, but I tried to ignore them and not let them bring me down. *Dr. Cole said it would be extremely rare for AFib to return. Calm down, it's not happening again. Wait and see until after the anniversary. I'm not ready for my heart to ruin another thing. If I get worse, I'll have to fly home to see my usual team of doctors.* I imagined returning to Boston, defeated. *My heart has to be better for at least a few years. I can't be sick again so soon. What's going on? I have to be strong enough now to be away from home for a long time. I don't want my heart to prevent me from continuing to work until the job ends in the fall.* As I was starting to live a fulfilling life away from the hospital, I wasn't ready to be thrust back into the life of tests, appointments, and disappointments.

Constantly thinking about the flutters made them worse as it had during my AFib episodes. I tried to stay busy and focus on the facts in order to calm myself down. *The flutters come and go but only occur inside my dorm room. Whenever I'm in there, I feel crummy. I get a lump in my throat. When I'm outside of my room, or at work, I feel fine.* I didn't know what to think as these types of symptoms were not what I had experienced before.

A few days later, at the morning meeting at work, we had a lesson about poisonous flowers. At the daily briefing we learned about monkshood, a flowering plant in Alaska also known as wolf's bane. It is a perennial herb with flowers that range in color from blue to dark purple. In late June, I picked this flower at a gas station because it was pretty, without knowing what it was. I kept the flower in a cup of water on my desk near my bed in my room. I touched the plant only on the day I picked it, but I was breathing the fumes it released every night as I slept. The flower had been in my room for one month.

After the briefing, I researched the symptoms associated with this specific type of flower poisoning, beyond what was discussed in the meeting. The first symptom of ingesting the flower is the rapid onset of life-threatening heart rhythm changes. Respiratory paralysis and abnormal heart rhythms can lead to death. This explained my heartbeat irregularities. Although I had touched the flower only once and had not ingested it, it was somehow making me sick. If I had not attended the meeting at work, I would have continued to think that my AFib had resumed. I immediately threw out the flower while wearing gloves, and never felt the flutters again. Focusing on the present, I stopped thinking about experiences from a year before.

My Surgeryversary Hike and the Savage Alpine Trail

Once my confidence returned, no longer feeling unwell, I decided to do something special to commemorate how far I had come in the year since the surgery. I contacted a hotel hiking guide and told her, "Take me on the most challenging hike you offer to guests!" On August 9th, exactly one year after my surgery, we embarked on a demanding hike in the wilderness, which had many steep hills and challenges. Called "Steps through Time," it spanned six miles. The title was fitting, and it was the most physically demanding activity I had undertaken in Alaska to date.

As we went along, the guide rated how grueling the hills would be on a "shitty" scale of one to ten. She also gave me some welcome warnings in advance of what we were facing. We'd laugh about the challenging times ahead instead of feeling apprehensive. I never wanted to quit when hiking, even though it was hot and the hills were steep. Sometimes I paused to look at the bright pink fireweed flowers or the smooth white birch trees along the way, hoping to catch a glimpse of an animal scurrying about. Although I was slow, panting and resting often, I made it to the hunter's cabin, the focal point of the hike. At the end of the six miles, we took photos, and I emailed them to my doctors. I was thrilled to show off how different my year had been compared to the previous ones. My care team was elated to see how well I was doing.

On August 15th, I went on another hike in Denali National Park, the Savage Alpine Trail, with a friend. The four-mile hike has a steep incline, with an elevation change of 1,200 feet. The surface is made up of compacted gravel and soil with stone steps along the path. My friend was not aware of my health history, but I warned him ahead of time that I needed to go at a slow pace. He was patient and we took our time with frequent rests. Going up in elevation was challenging for me, but he didn't mind waiting, and we had a great time together enjoying all the sights along the way.

We reached a large rock after climbing high up the trail. Along the way, we saw a pika, a cute furry animal like a rabbit. That made the journey worthwhile, although it was raining on and off and visibility wasn't great. Instead of completing the hike and climbing to 1,200 feet, my friend and I decided to come down from the rock. When we descended, we couldn't find the trail we had come up on and needed to walk wherever we could find safe footing. The rain created some slick spots, but we made it down through all of the rocks and gravel on the steep decline. We had to wing it; it was a white-knuckle experience, and we were lucky we didn't get hurt.

After the hike, we decided we wanted to do more in the park before returning to the village, so we walked around the Savage River. To reach the road where the shuttle bus stopped to take us home, we took what we thought was a shortcut off the trail. We needed to climb up a steep, rocky, brush-packed hill to reach the roadway. In Denali National Park, there are no rules about staying exclusively on trails, and you can walk wherever the mood takes you. Seeing the path ahead, my friend suggested, "Let's turn back and find an easier way up to the street."

I shook my head. "No way!" I didn't actually know how steep the hill was. It was deceiving when it appeared so close, and I wanted to keep trying. "We're going to do it," I naively stated.

With a set time we had to be on the roadway in order to catch the bus, I couldn't stop to rest and needed to power through the challenging hike. My friend and I whacked away at the brush and climbed up the steep hill. Just before reaching the top, I dropped to my hands and knees to crawl through the dirt, plants, and sharp gravel for the final few feet, since the hill was too steep for me to stand and walk up. I was ecstatic when I made it to the top and onto the roadway ahead of the bus. *I've never done anything so demanding! That was much harder than my surgeryversary hike. I couldn't have previously accomplished that. If I can do that, there's no telling what else I can do.* For the first time, I saw what my new heart and I could do if I pushed myself. My friend and I even went on an additional hike prior to returning to the village, making it a three-hike day, including the very steep hill.

Benjamin Climbs 1,000 Feet

A month later, on my last day in the park, September 13th, I accomplished an extremely taxing hike. I completed the Alpine Trail Hike, which was far more grueling than any other I had done. The trail is only 0.8 miles but ascends 1,010 feet in that short distance. It took me an hour each way, up and down. The weather was warm, the elevation was high, and the ascent was terribly steep. Many times, the old feeling of wanting to quit returned. *Keep resting,* I thought as I fell behind my friends. *Don't go back to your old ways and give up. You don't have to race to the top and you're safe on your own. Your friends are right there, and they can see you.*

Upon reaching the top of the trail, I had an unobstructed, full view of Mt. Denali. None of the usual clouds in the sky interfered. Aside from the view from my small-plane ride, I had never seen the mountain from so high up. I was out of breath and sat down to rest for a while. After resting, I fully comprehended what I had accomplished. I took in my surroundings and could see for miles. *This view's cool, but it's more exciting that I completed the hike!* After a short amount of further hiking, my friends and I went back down the Alpine Trail. It was much easier than the way up, but I still needed to be remarkably careful with my footing on the rocky path.

When I returned to the village, I emailed my family to tell them what I had done. I titled my email, *Benjamin climbed 1,000 feet!* Mom replied, "Benjamin, you are amazing!" I felt amazing too. Some of the best photos I have of myself in Alaska were taken on top of that trail.

Returning Home

At the end of September, I returned home to Boston. On my first night back at my parents' house, when I returned from the airport, I had my picture taken in front of the Alaska poster at the dining room table. Feeling more like an Alaskan than a Bostonian, I proudly smiled in the picture while remembering all I had accomplished.

Although I was becoming a skilled hiker, I accepted that I still had my limits in Alaska. The elevation prevented me from running. When I was back in Boston, I was uncertain of my fitness level. In early October, I went for my first run since May. I ran 2.5 miles, and I couldn't believe it. Owing to my lack of practice, I had assumed my endurance would suffer, but I did better than my usual training runs before Alaska. The same month, my friends welcomed me back with open arms as I rejoined the run club. I commenced training for the next B.A.A. 5K.

Before I moved to Alaska, I read on the Denali National Park Facebook page, "Sometimes the trail ahead of us is not clear or obvious, but that makes the journey all the more successful in the end!" It's so true. I had an amazing time and discovered the capabilities of my body. Alaska taught me I could try anything. Back at home, I decided to keep adventuring and living life to the fullest. I am now much more receptive to opportunities that come my way since I don't know when my abilities may decline. While I am still able, I must take advantage of everything and actively seek out new and challenging opportunities.

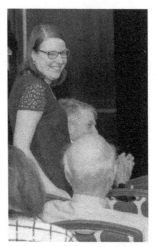

Emily at Dr. Washington's Talk
(October 10, 2018)

Realizing an Opportunity to Help

During my last weeks in Alaska, Dr. Washington emailed me and told me he was giving a fundraising talk to MGH donors. He inquired, "Can I feature you in my presentation? If so, can you please send me pictures from the race and from your time spent in Alaska to use during my talk?"

"Of course," I replied and sent him pictures to use. About a month after I returned to Boston, my family and I were invited to a local hotel for the speech.

The night began when I met one of the fundraising coordinators. She shook my hand saying eagerly, "Thank you for allowing Dr. Washington to tell your incredible story." It set the scene for what was to come. Prior to the talk, I was ushered into the ballroom to speak privately with Dr. Washington. I had not seen him in over a year since my last postop appointment. It felt nice to see him in a relaxed setting. We caught up and reviewed what he planned to say about me, making sure I was comfortable with him disclosing my history. My family and the donors came into the room a while later.

Dr. Washington's presentation was titled "Successes and Challenges in Adult Congenital Heart Disease." He explained that there have been seventy-five years of progress with congenital heart disease (CHD). More adults live with CHD than children, since symptoms can go unrecognized in children and manifest at an older age. The care of patients like me required multidisciplinary teams for optimal management. He spoke about other cardiac patients and then he arrived at my story.

The slide about me was called "A very special MGH patient ..." It included a diagram illustrating my heart condition and detailed some of my history. He introduced me, saying, "We have an amazing person here tonight. ... Emily is thirty-six years old and she was born with a very, very unusual heart problem." He explained his diagram and the issues in the structure of my heart. After detailing my history at the hospital, he went on to recount some of my struggles.

The slides advanced to one titled "We are proud of you, Emily!" This slide had a still picture from my television interview after the 5K race and a picture of me taken on top of the hill in front of Mt. Denali on my last hike in the park. He concluded his talk by saying, "Emily has really done us proud. ... She is clearly able to do things she wasn't able to before. ... Emily's recovery was in large part due to her determination to get back on track and have a normal life."

It was nice to be recognized by Dr. Washington and hear my story told. When he pointed me out in the audience, I stood up, smiled, and waved to the large room full of people. Most of the attendees were older and smiled back at me while clapping. I sat back down, feeling good and not self-conscious about what I had done.

Afterward, many attendees came up to speak with me. They told me they were inspired by my story and called me a hero, to my bewilderment. *I don't get it. All I did was go on living and trying.* Mom took me aside and said, "A hero is someone who inspires others to do well. You fit the bill in a thousand categories." *I don't know if I feel that way, but it's nice to hear.*

Audience member remarks could be odd, such as those from one person who said, "You look like you have great color," or the person who saw me drinking wine and said, shocked, "You can drink?!" I'm used to strange comments, and I let them roll off my back most of the time. These didn't faze me as I'd heard them many times before.

One person said, "Congratulations on your good luck." My path has been a combination of good luck, the tremendous expertise of all the doctors and care teams coming together to do their best for me, and, of course, all the support my family and friends have given me throughout the years. All the pieces working together helped create the best outcome for me. I worked hard to achieve new things, but without all of these people in my life, I couldn't have gotten to where I am today.

Perhaps the best comment of the night came from an older gentleman. He came up to me and asked me, "How do you feel now?"

"I feel so much better and my heart's improved," I said.

He responded, "Why the hell didn't they do this sooner?" I laughed at his response for a solid minute.

Although it wouldn't have been the right time to do the surgery prior to experiencing AFib, his sentiment was exactly right, and it was great to hear. It was something stated so plainly and was so obvious now that everything had worked out.

I texted Mabel during the event and asked her, "Why's it such a big deal and why are people calling me a hero?"

She responded, "I know for us it's just stuff we've always dealt with and getting through illness is not a choice. To them, you're their hero because of your perseverance. Remember, doctors go into medicine to help people and you're thriving. You ran a 5K and then were like 'Bye, I'm going to Alaska.' It's amazing!" All of Mabel's thoughtful comments sank in sometime later after the buzz of the evening wore off.

At the end of the night Dr. Washington spoke with me. "No patients have ever come to a donor event. You put a special touch on the evening." He smiled and we said our goodbyes, and I hoped I had helped in some way. On the walk to the subway on the way home, my family members thanked me for inviting them to the talk. When Dad hesitated over what to thank me for, I joked he should say, "Thank you for not dying!" He laughed and agreed. It was a perfect night.

That same night I received a job offer to work at another university in Boston in the HR department. Despite a continuing interest in pursuing a less traditional career, I accepted the job. I thought I should consider what Sam often said to me: "You don't have to go away on vacation to be happy. You have to make the most of the place where you are." I could accept the job security and at the same time keep my options wide open and limitless for my future.

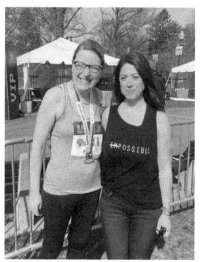

Emily and Mabel, After the Race (April 14, 2018)

Reflections

On the subway one day, I saw a bandaged man speaking with his daughter on their way home from the hospital. She was barking directions at him to make sure he'd get home safely: "Don't pretend you're all right, call me."

"How do you pretend to be okay?" he asked her.

That's a strange question. How do you not know how to pretend to be okay when ill? How can you not have the skills to hide a problem and to carry on as though everything's okay? As an adult, I haven't had much time off from being ill. Starting with my glaucoma diagnosis at age twenty-eight, to AFib at almost age thirty-one, through the second heart surgery when I was thirty-five, I never got a break from major health events. To have had many stable years and then eight bad years in succession was tough, and I often pretended I was fine, even when my body was falling apart.

Illness gave me an excuse to stop engaging in life. *I'm doing so well I don't need to be disengaged anymore. I don't have to pretend I'm okay, because for now, I am. Remember, you don't have to limit yourself in the same ways anymore. This might take practice. I treasure the predictability of health. I won't have it forever, but I love having it for as long as it lasts.*

Adjust to New Possibilities

Oftentimes when I tried something new, Mom asked, "Are you sure you can do that?"

"Yes, don't worry anymore," I said back. "I know your instinct is to worry, but you don't have to so much or about the same things. We all have to adjust to this new life I have."

"You might have died after running the 5K," Sam said.

"Not everything's so scary anymore," I responded. "No one ever said that was a risk for me. Remember what Mabel said to you, Mom, when she found out I was going to Alaska, 'Emily's always up for an adventure.' Think of it like that." *I like that other people see me this way. I want to feel adventurous. I don't have to control everything.* "I never do anything that's crazy or reckless on purpose."

In a way, the surgery caused my body to start over. It's like everything reset and started working again. My weight has stayed stable, and I no longer get frequent colds. At times I forget I am changed and I go back to sitting on the couch, watching TV, doing nothing meaningful. *Doing nothing sounds great.* Then I think, *time's ticking away. I don't know how much time I have in a body that works so well. I have more energy than I think. I don't need as many rests. Keep going, don't stop. Whatever I can do, even if it's small, is a win.* I get up off the couch and play my favorite songs and dance, do jumping jacks, or run in place. *See, I can still do more than ever before.*

At my weekly run club, I challenge myself to keep up with the fastest runners in the club when they sprint. We all stand on the starting line and take off at the same time. *Keep going! I know I can do this at least 100 meters.* I stop when I have to, breathless and in need of a rest; the others keep going, but for those few seconds when I am keeping up, it's like a dream. I am constantly learning, not merely what I can do, but how noncardiac patients feel with healthy hearts.

Chronic Illness or Injury

During a visit to Japan in 2009, Sam and I took the subway after a long, hot day shopping and touring the sites in Tokyo. When we got onto the train, I was sweating, with a red face, and was tired from a day of exertion and carrying bags. *I'm so tired, I just want to sit down.* I limply grabbed onto a pole to hang on and glanced at the glass window above a row of seats. There to my shock and surprise was a sticker depicting the usual priority seats for elderly and pregnant people, but *also* seats for people with heart conditions. The sign had nondescript human figures, one with a large belly, one with a cane, and one with a heart highlighted in the center of their chest. *I've never seen a sign like this anywhere!* I triumphantly sat down in this special seat without any guilt, happy my condition was being understood and recognized. *I don't have to ask for it or prove I need it by having something obvious that shows my illness. It feels like someone knows about what I go through. It's so rare. I'm glad it was done in a non-demeaning way.*

When I see signs in public about heart conditions, they are usually about cautioning people not to participate in activities, like climbing a staircase or going on a ride at a theme park. One summer, Mabel and I went on a hike in the woods in upstate New York. We reached the pinnacle of the hike, a water tower with steps up to see the view of the valley below. At the bottom of the stairs a sign cautioned, "Do not use staircase if you have a heart condition." Infuriated, I stood at the bottom of the staircase. "I can't stand this. Who's to say we can't do this? There's nothing here describing which kind of heart condition is affected by the activity and what might happen if we try." *All cardiac survivors are different. We can all do different things and activities affect us differently.*

"I'm sure it's to protect from liability," Mabel said. "I think it would make more sense for a sign to describe the challenge, like steep climb ahead or high elevation increase. Warning to those with heart conditions."

"You're right, that makes sense," I replied. "I hiked up the mountain to get to the water tower, so what makes the sign maker think I can't also go up these stairs?"

"It's stupid," Mabel said. "I can go up and let you know what I see. I don't think there's a risk for me if I go."

"I'll stay down here. I don't care enough to go."

Mabel went up the tower.

I wish more information was available and understood about invisible illnesses, I thought as I waited for her return. *If the signs were more descriptive there could be more inclusion rather than blanket exclusion.*

Accepting Imperfection

Since I was born with a chronic condition, I've never thought about a life when I'll be cured. I appreciate what I can do. I don't know what a "healthy" body feels like, so I don't truly know what I'm missing. Even with limitations, there's always a way. Modifications will allow me to do some of what I long to do.

My body will forever betray me in one way or another and will never be "perfect" or "healthy." Even if I live the healthiest life possible, eating all the right foods, exercising, and living in a bubble, health conditions still occur.

Once again, *Grey's Anatomy* imparted some wisdom on this predicament in life. In the episode "We Didn't Start the Fire," a main character who developed a heart condition later in life said to her friend, "I have a heart that I no longer trust. I live day by day trying to get it to not blow up again and hoping that the fix they gave me stays a fix."[9] I sat on the couch thinking about this statement. *I agree, I dread the day when my body falls apart again. I'll get through it, but I don't want it to happen.*

Objectivity

In 2019, I was at my annual gynecological exam with my new doctor, at our first appointment together. I lay calmly on the table, and she said, "There will be some pressure now and it won't hurt much."

I replied, "I know, it's not a big deal."

The doctor responded, laughing, "Compared to open-heart surgery, I guess, no, it's not."

"Actually, needles in the eye are worse," I said. *I'm not trying to be funny. It's true.*

My doctor said, "I know you're tough."

Her response got me thinking. *People think I am tough, strong, and brave for going through open-heart surgery, but nurses, aides, and doctors got me through surgeries. My body healed on its own. My strong immune system did its job and my heart muscle recovered, making me gradually better. I didn't have to think about it. There might be pain with surgery and procedures, but I can take pills to manage that. The memory of pain fades with time.*

I left the doctor's office and continued to think during my subway ride home. *It's other stuff that's more problematic. A big problem that I know is coming is not as hard as incremental things over a long period of time, like my slowly developing a cataract, and unexpected small irritations like burning MRIs. No one can get me through those by telling me how to cope with them. They haven't experienced them first hand and can't really explain what to expect or how they will feel.*

I thought back to some challenging times when I waited at Dr. Knight's office for an eye-pressure reading. I used to have to text Sam for a pep talk. I'd get so nervous waiting to hear what my eye pressure would be that the positive encouragement was helpful. It was never the tests making me nervous; it was figuring out what to do if I received bad news and had to make treatment decisions.

Stay objective. See both sides of the argument. Should I take my inflammation drop because it helps with the pain, or should I skip it because it makes my cataract worse? My eye will require more surgery in the future, and this will speed that up. Make a pro and con list. Family and friends will always be emotional about medical struggles. What is objectively best for me? Focus on the options to solve the crises and the parts you can control.

Embrace the Positives

Oh no, I can't see the words on the paper! There's a cloud in my vision. My eye's worse. Did my glaucoma worsen overnight? I panicked and took my glasses off. Suddenly my vision was clear. *Oh ... It's just a smudge on the lens.*

I often think to myself when my fears creep in, *my conditions will probably return or get worse. It could be anything, not just my heart or eye. I can get through it. I've gotten through everything else. There will always be something good with the negative, even if I don't know what it is yet.*

Move Forward

Dr. Cole told me at our fall 2018 appointment, about a year after the heart surgery, "You weren't in good shape before the surgery. Your health is much better now so you should keep exploring, trying new things and don't worry."

That's hard. Stop waiting each day for another medical disaster? How am I gonna do that? But maybe she's right. I'll remember what I didn't do or try and regret what I missed. Something negative might happen, but it might be worth doing anyway.

I recognize now, after the valve replacement was so successful, if there are solutions to my predicaments that can improve the time I have left, I should try them. When I contemplate dying young or becoming ill in the future, I say to myself, *it's not always going to be my turn. It'll be someone else's turn to be sick and then it'll be mine. For now, I'm going to enjoy this healthy period. Other people are going through much worse and conquer their own battles every day.* Thinking about that helps me to keep moving forward and to never give up.

Fearing Death

Some people are worried about dying. Mabel and I discussed it on the phone.

I said, "Dying doesn't affect me. I'll be dead. It mostly affects the people left behind."

"Yes, that's true, I guess," she said.

"Death can be taboo and hard to talk about. But it's always been a known variable in my life," I said. "There's no need to fear death unless there's family and friends who depend on you, who you worry about leaving behind."

"I'm not sure I agree," Mabel replied. "I've always been very afraid of the idea of dying. I want to live."

"I think the hard stuff in life is living with long-term illness or unmanageable pain."

"Well, I believe in compassionate care if someone has a terminal illness, but I've never thought of congenital heart defects as a terminal illness. We have treatment and options and choices of how we want to tackle these things."

"Yeah, but having faced death and long-term incurable illness, I think there are worse events than dying, like suffering a major accident or mental trauma."

"People live through terrible traumas and find ways to push through. There's still so many things that can be enjoyed in life, even if it's not what you pictured."

Communication

Everyone will probably experience being ill at least once. Most of the population is temporarily abled for the majority of their lifetime. Mabel and I texted about this topic.

"Why are illnesses such a secret? Why can't most people talk openly without feeling shame?" I asked her.

"I don't know. I've always tried to talk about it, but you haven't. Now you're starting to," Mabel said.

I responded, "We didn't make ourselves sick on purpose. It's the hand we were dealt. It could be a genetic disease or by chance, but it's scary to talk about. There's so much judgment and strange preconceived notions. When I told someone once about you they asked me if you have an unusual gait. I have no idea why! They know I don't and why they think you would makes no sense. Or why someone with a cardiac condition in general would is so odd."

"The internet's changing everything. People post about all this stuff now. You never talked about your problems before and might've needed medical help. Now after the surgery, when you're pretty sure you won't have any problems, you start sharing it. I find that interesting," Mabel typed.

"Yeah and I don't think I would've asked for help before either. I would've tried to handle my problems on my own. Maybe, also, I feel like it's not such a risk that I'll be treated differently now. And I've been practicing how to communicate about my condition, to make people understand."

"The more people share their stories and learn about other people's struggles, the less ignorant people will be," she typed.

"You never know, I guess. The next person I tell might know someone with a similar condition or actually have it themselves."

Remaining Resilient

Before I moved to Alaska, Dr. Cole mentioned that MGH wanted to feature me on their ACHD webpage. While I was in Alaska I was interviewed, and after Thanksgiving the article was published.

I thought as I read it, *I'm glad they highlighted my childhood memories and time spent in the hospital. They did a good job describing my relationship with the doctors.*

What Emily values most about this team is that they are just as confident in her as she is in them. "When I feel like something is wrong, they never doubt me, and I never doubt them. I know they can find a way to fix it or to manage it," says Emily. Emily knows that her valve will be replaced in the future, but she doesn't allow that to stop her from doing the things she loves, like traveling, hiking and running. "All of my conditions can be treated, but they cannot be cured," she says. "But after each surgery, I will have a period of years where I feel this good, and I'm going to take advantage of it!"[10]

This really shows what I want to show the world: positivity and determination.

After all of the special events, I finally took in everything that happened over the previous year. Thinking back to all of the positive comments I received from sharing my story in the television interview after the race, at Dr. Washington's talk, and in the MGH website article made me think, *how can I continue to tell the world about my experiences and help empower others? I also want to motivate doctors and caregivers not to give up on us patients.*

I didn't do anything special. I didn't try harder than anyone else. I had no choice in any of this. But people are inspired by my success. Sometimes it's difficult to see how much you affect and inspire other people because you're living your life the best way you know how. A friend recently disclosed their own health condition to me and instead of saying, "I had cancer," they said, "I am a cancer survivor."

How striking. I would never say I'm a heart attack or heart surgery survivor. I always say I have a heart condition even though I'm a survivor, too. Maybe I should say this as part of my introduction. I should be proud I've made it through these trying life events.

The Finish Line

I've run to the home plate in softball, to the hospital entrance before surgery, to the nurse's desk after surgery, to the finish line in a 5K, and to adventures in Alaska. Now I have to run into my future, facing challenges and sticking with my innate perseverance.

Before my second surgery, I used to describe my limitations as having to avoid endurance activities or lifting heavy weights. I never tried to push those boundaries, readily sitting on the sidelines. But now, I no longer have a rehearsed explanation when I'm asked, because my possibilities are endless. I can try anything with modifications.

Sam recently said, "Anyone who runs in a race is an athlete." That's a powerful way to think about myself now. After my successful 5K race, I am still trying new endeavors because I never know what I can do. What I've learned is there will always be ups and downs, yet through them all, I'll just try!

Now this athlete's signing off to go for a run and find a new finish line!

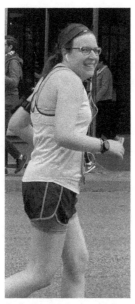

Emily, Age 39, During the Race
(April 16, 2022)

Acknowledgments

This book would not be possible without all of the support I received from my family, friends, and doctors. Thank you for all that you have done, all you will do, and your encouragement.

To MF, thank you for staying up nights and weekends to help me edit the book. When you're right, you're right! I can't thank you enough for all of the time you took to help me. To Mom, Dad, and MW, thank you for being there through all of my ups and downs and providing me advice, editing, and copy to make this book a success.

NS, you are my best friend forever! I couldn't have made it through the years without you and your constant support. I value our friendship more than anything and all of your insights and edits have been immensely helpful.

Thank you to all of my doctors and nurses past and present who have kept me alive and thriving.

SS in the Writing Center helped me edit the book and rewrite it until it made sense. I am grateful for all of your advice and help.

For my book doula, Anna Jaworski, thank you for everything. I couldn't have done it without your coaching and wisdom.

To my editor, Michael Sims, thank you for shaping the book up to be the best it can be. It's much better with all of your suggestions and edits.

My graphic artist, Helen Gao, made the book enticing and designed the cover and interior beautifully.

KZ, I couldn't have figured out copyright and the glossary without you. Thank you.

Medical Glossary

Arrhythmia   A problem with the rate or rhythm of your heartbeat. It means that your heart beats too quickly, too slowly, or with an irregular pattern.

Atrial fibrillation   The most common type of arrhythmia. The cause is a disorder in the heart's electrical system. ... The electrical impulse of the heart is not regular. This is because the sinoatrial node no longer controls the heart rhythm.

Atrial flutter   In atrial flutter, the ventricles (lower heart chambers) may beat very rapidly, but in a regular pattern.

Cardiac ablation procedure   A procedure that is used to scar small areas in your heart that may be involved in your heart rhythm problems. This can prevent the abnormal electrical signals or rhythms from moving through the heart. During the procedure, small wires called electrodes are placed inside your heart to measure your heart's electrical activity. When the source of the problem is found, the tissue causing the problem is destroyed.

Cardioversion   A method to bring an abnormal heart rhythm back to normal. ... Electrical cardioversion is done with a device that gives off an electrical shock to the heart to change the rhythm back to normal.

Catheterization procedure   Involves passing a thin flexible tube (catheter) into the right or left side of the heart ... inserted from the groin or the arm ... placed into a vein or artery in your leg or arm. ... The doctor can measure pressure and blood flow in the heart's chambers and in the large arteries around the heart.

Congestive heart failure   Heart failure means that your heart can't pump enough oxygen-rich blood to meet your body's needs. Heart failure doesn't mean that your heart has stopped or is about to stop beating. But without enough blood flow, your organs may not work well, which can cause serious problems.

Echocardiogram (Echo)   A test that uses sound waves to create pictures of the heart.

Electrocardiogram (ECG or EKG)   A test that records the electrical activity of the heart.

Heart attack/myocardial infarction   A heart attack happens when blood flow to the heart suddenly becomes blocked. Without the blood coming in, the heart can't get oxygen. If not treated quickly, the heart muscle begins to die.

Incentive spirometer/deep breathing exerciser   An instrument for measuring the air capacity of the lungs.

Leaflets   A flap of a valve of a heart or blood vessel.

Left coronary artery   Carries blood to the heart muscle.

Maze surgery   Treats atrial fibrillation with small cuts in the heart muscle. The cuts form scars that make a path for the heart's electrical signals.

Mitral stenosis   A disorder in which the mitral valve does not fully open. This restricts the flow of blood.

Mitral valve   One of the four valves in your heart. Heart valves have flaps that open and close. The flaps make sure that blood flows in the right direction through your heart and to the rest of your body. When your heart beats, the flaps open to let blood through. Between heartbeats they close to stop the blood from flowing backward. The mitral valve opens to let blood flow from your heart's upper left chamber to the lower left chamber. When the lower left chamber contracts (squeezes) to pump blood to your body, the mitral valve closes tightly to keep any blood from flowing backward.

Mitral valve regurgitation   A disorder in which the mitral valve on the left side of the heart does not close properly. Regurgitation means leaking from a valve that does not close all the way.

Palpitation   Feelings or sensations that your heart is pounding or racing. They can be felt in your chest, throat, or neck.

PICC line (Peripherally inserted central catheter)   A tube that goes into a vein in your arm. It helps carry nutrients or medicine into your body. It is also used to take blood when you need to have blood tests.

Pilonidal cyst   A pocket that forms around a hair follicle in the crease between the buttocks.

Pulmonary artery   The main artery to the lungs.

Transesophageal echocardiogram   The sonographer will ... insert a small tube into the ... esophagus. The end of the tube contains a device to send out sound waves. The sound waves reflect off the structures in the heart and are displayed on a screen as images of the heart and blood vessels. Because the esophagus is right behind the heart, this method is used to get clearer pictures of the heart.

Ventricular fibrillation   Severely abnormal heart rhythm (arrhythmia) that is life threatening. When it occurs in the lower chambers of the heart, it is called VF.

Notes

1. NIH U.S. National Library of Medicine. *Anomalous left coronary artery from the pulmonary artery.* A.D.A.M., Inc. 05 Jan. 2021. Web. 08 Feb 2021. Available at: https://medlineplus.gov/ency/article/007323.htm

2. Adult Congenital Heart Association. *ACHA Announces Funding of Organization's Inaugural Research Grants.* 01 May 2019. Web. 08 Feb 2021. https://www.achaheart.org/about-us/news/2019/acha-announces-funding-of-organization-s-inaugural-research-grants/

3. Rodriguez-Gonzalez, Moises, MD, Antonio Moruno Tirado, MD, Reza Hosseinpour, MD, Jose Santos de Soto, MD. "Anomalous Origin of the Left Coronary Artery from the Pulmonary Artery: Diagnoses and Surgical Results in 12 Pediatric Patients." *Tex Heart Inst J.* 2015 Aug; 42(4): 350–356. 2015 Aug 1. Web. Available at: https://www.ncbi.nlm.nih.gov/pmc/articles/PMC4567127/

4. Peña, Elena, Elsie T. Nguyen, Naeem Merchant, Carole Dennie. "ALCAPA Syndrome: Not Just a Pediatric Disease." *RadioGraphics*, Vol. 29, No. 2, 01 Mar 2009. Web. Available at: https://pubs.rsna.org/doi/full/10.1148/rg.292085059

5. Boston Children's Hospital. "Anomalous Left Coronary Artery from the Pulmonary Artery (ALCAPA)." Web. 27 Feb 2023. Available at: https://www.childrenshospital.org/conditions/anomalous-left-coronary-artery-pulmonary-artery-alcapa

6. "Edward J. Madden Open Hearts Camp," About. 2015 Madden Hearts Camp. n.d. Web. 08 Feb 2021. https://www.openheartscamp.org/about-us-2/

7. *Grey's Anatomy:* Season 2, Episode 27. Losing My Religion 15 May 2006 Director: Mark Tinker Writers: Shonda Rhimes.

8. *Grey's Anatomy:* Season 2, Episode 27. Losing My Religion 15 May 2006 Director: Mark Tinker Writers: Shonda Rhimes.

9. *Grey's Anatomy:* Season 15, Episode 15. We Didn't Start the Fire. 28 Feb 2019. Director: Chandra Wilson. Writer: Andy Reaser.

10. "Patient Story: Emily." *Mass General Hospital.* 28 Nov 2018. Web. 12 Dec 2020. Available at: https://www.massgeneral.org/heartcenter/news/newsarticle.aspx?id=6959.

Sources

CDC; Materials developed by CDC. Reference to specific commercial products, manufacturers, companies, or trademarks does not constitute its endorsement or recommendation by the U.S. Government, Department of Health and Human Services, or Centers for Disease Control and Prevention.

MedlinePlus, National Library of Medicine

Wiktionary

About the Author

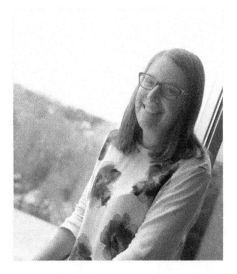

Emily Falcon lives in Massachusetts. At seven weeks old, she had a heart attack and was diagnosed with anomalous origin of the left coronary artery from the pulmonary artery (ALCAPA). This led to two open-heart surgeries, one at age six and another at age thirty-five. She loves travel and animals, both of which have helped her get through difficult times. While living a constrained life, Emily has sought out adventures whenever she can, such as trekking up volcanoes to observe mountain gorillas in Uganda, volunteering with cheetahs and baboons in Namibia, playing with wolves at the Arctic Circle, and eating with orangutans in Singapore. She is now an athlete who participates in a weekly run club and runs in 5K races throughout the year. She hopes to inspire others with health limitations to never waste a moment and not let life pass them by.

She can be emailed at dont.waste.a.second.press@gmail.com.